T0227168

Victims of Abuse

Guest Editor

SHARON W. STARK, PhD, RN, APN-C, CFN

NURSING CLINICS
OF NORTH AMERICA

www.nursing.theclinics.com

Consulting Editor
SUZANNE S. PREVOST, PhD, RN, COI

December 2011 • Volume 46 • Number 4

SAUNDERS an imprint of ELSEVIER, Inc.

W.B. SAUNDERS COMPANY

A Division of Elsevier Inc.

1600 John F. Kennedy Blvd., Suite 1800 ● Philadelphia, PA 19103-2899

http://www.theclinics.com

NURSING CLINICS OF NORTH AMERICA Volume 46, Number 4
December 2011 ISSN 0029-6465, ISBN-13: 978-1-4557-7986-4

Editor: Katie Hartner
Developmental Editor: Donald Mumford

© **2011 Elsevier Inc. All rights reserved.**

This journal and the individual contributions contained in it are protected under copyright by Elsevier, and the following terms and conditions apply to their use:

Photocopying
Single photocopies of single articles may be made for personal use as allowed by national copyright laws. Permission of the Publisher and payment of a fee is required for all other photocopying, including multiple or systematic copying, copying for advertising or promotional purposes, resale, and all forms of document delivery. Special rates are available for educational institutions that wish to make photocopies for non-profit educational classroom use. For information on how to seek permission visit www.elsevier.com/permissions or call: (+44) 1865 843830 (UK)/ (+1) 215 239 3804 (USA).

Derivative Works
Subscribers may reproduce tables of contents or prepare lists of articles including abstracts for internal circulation within their institutions. Permission of the Publisher is required for resale or distribution outside the institution. Permission of the Publisher is required for all other derivative works, including compilations and translations (please consult www.elsevier.com/permissions).

Electronic Storage or Usage
Permission of the Publisher is required to store or use electronically any material contained in this journal, including any article or part of an article (please consult www.elsevier.com/permissions). Except as outlined above, no part of this publication may be reproduced, stored in a retrieval system or transmitted in any form or by any means, electronic, mechanical, photocopying, recording or otherwise, without prior written permission of the Publisher.

Notice
No responsibility is assumed by the Publisher for any injury and/or damage to persons or property as a matter of products liability, negligence or otherwise, or from any use or operation of any methods, products, instructions or ideas contained in the material herein. Because of rapid advances in the medical sciences, in particular, independent verification of diagnoses and drug dosages should be made.

Although all advertising material is expected to conform to ethical (medical) standards, inclusion in this publication does not constitute a guarantee or endorsement of the quality or value of such product or of the claims made of it by its manufacturer.

Nursing Clinics of North America (ISSN 0029-6465) is published quarterly by Elsevier Inc., 360 Park Avenue South, New York, NY 10010-1710. Months of issue are March, June, September, and December. Periodicals postage paid at New York, NY and additional mailing offices. Subscription price per year is, $144.00 (US individuals), $360.00 (US institutions), $260.00 (international individuals), $440.00 (international institutions), $210.00 (Canadian individuals), $440.00 (Canadian institutions), $79.00 (US students), and $129.00 (international students). To receive student/resident rate, orders must be accompanied by name of affiliated institution, date of term, and the signature of program/residency coordinator on institution letterhead. Orders will be billed at individual rate until proof of status is received. Foreign air speed delivery is included in all *Clinics* subscription prices. All prices are subject to change without notice. **POSTMASTER:** Send address changes to *Nursing Clinics*, Elsevier Health Sciences Division, Subscription Customer Service, 3251 Riverport Lane, Maryland Heights, MO 63043. **Customer Service: Telephone: 1-800-654-2452** (U.S. and Canada); **1-314-447-8871 (outside U.S. and Canada). Fax: 1-314-447-8029. E-mail: journalscustomerservice-usa@elsevier.com** (for print support) and **journalsonlinesupport-usa@elsevier.com** (for online support).

Nursing Clinics of North America is covered in *EMBASE/Excerpta Medica, MEDLINE/PubMed (Index Medicus), Social Sciences Citation Index, Current Contents, ASCA, Cumulative Index to Nursing, RNdex Top 100,* and Allied Health Literature and International Nursing Index (INI).

Printed and bound by CPI Group (UK) Ltd, Croydon, CR0 4YY

Transferred to Digital Print 2011

Contributors

CONSULTING EDITOR

SUZANNE S. PREVOST, PhD, RN, COI
Associate Dean, Practice and Community Engagement, University of Kentucky, Lexington, Kentucky

GUEST EDITOR

SHARON W. STARK, PhD, RN, APN-C, CFN
Associate Dean, Forensic Nursing and Nurse Practitioner Programs Coordinator, Monmouth University, Marjorie K. Unterberg School of Nursing and Health Studies, West Long Branch, New Jersey

AUTHORS

SUSAN ARAUJO, RN, MSN, NE-BC
Director of Patient Care, Community Medical Center, Toms River, New Jersey

NARGIS ASAD, PhD
Assistant Professor, Department of Psychiatry, The Aga Khan University Hospital, Karachi, Pakistan

JEANETTE M. DALY, RN, PhD
Associate Research Scientist, Department of Family Medicine, Carver College of Medicine, University of Iowa, Iowa City, Iowa

CIRA FRASER, PhD, RN, ACNS-BC
Associate Professor and Graduate Faculty, Monmouth University, Marjorie K. Unterberg School of Nursing and Health Studies, West Long Branch, New Jersey

KELSEY L. HEGARTY, PhD
Associate Professor, Department of General Practice, General Practice and Primary Health Care Academic Centre, University of Melbourne, Carlton, Victoria, Australia

SHELA AKBAR ALI HIRANI, MSN
Senior Instructor, School of Nursing, Aga Khan University, Karachi, Pakistan

SAIMA SHAMS HIRANI, MSN, RN
Senior Instructor, School of Nursing, Aga Khan University, Karachi, Pakistan

LAURA JANNONE, EdD, RN, NJ-CSN
Associate Professor, Coordinator of the School Nurse Program; Director, Nursing Graduate Programs, Monmouth University, Marjorie K. Unterberg School of Nursing and Health Studies, West Long Branch, New Jersey

ROZINA KARMALIANI, PhD, RN
Associate Professor, School of Nursing and Department of Community Health Sciences, Aga Khan University, Karachi, Pakistan

LAURA KELLY, PhD, PMHNP
Associate Professor, Monmouth University, Marjorie K. Unterberg School of Nursing and Health Studies, West Long Branch, New Jersey

ROSE KNAPP, DNP, RN, APN-C
Assistant Professor of Nursing, Monmouth University, Marjorie K. Unterberg School of Nursing and Health Studies, West Long Branch, New Jersey

JANET MAHONEY, RN, PhD, APN, ENA-BC
Monmouth University, Marjorie K. Unterberg School of Nursing and Health Studies, West Long Branch, New Jersey

JUDITH MCFARLANE, DrPH, RN, FAAN
Professor, Texas Woman's University, Nelda C. Stark College of Nursing, Houston, Texas

SHIREEN SHEHZAD, BScN
Senior Instructor, School of Nursing, Aga Khan University, Karachi, Pakistan

LAURA SOFIELD, RN, MSN, APN
Advanced Practice Nurse, Mid-Atlantic Geriatrics Association, Ocean, New Jersey

SHARON W. STARK, PhD, RN, APN-C, CFN
Associate Dean, Forensic Nursing and Nurse Practitioner Programs Coordinator, Monmouth University, Marjorie K. Unterberg School of Nursing and Health Studies, West Long Branch, New Jersey

LENE SYMES, PhD, RN
Associate Professor, Texas Woman's University, College of Nursing, Houston, Texas

MARYANN TROIANO, DNP, RN, APRN
Assistant Professor, Monmouth University, Marjorie K. Unterberg School of Nursing and Health Studies, West Long Branch, New Jersey

Contents

Preface   ix

Sharon W. Stark

Types of Abuse   385

Janet Mahoney

> The four most common types of abuse are physical, sexual, emotional, and economic. Abuse is often further categorized into child abuse, intimate partner violence, and elder abuse. This article describes the important role that nurses and health care providers play in detecting, assessing, and reporting abuse. Armed with increased knowledge about signs and symptoms of abuse, nurses can guide patients to the appropriate resources.

Abuse Across the Lifespan: Prevalence, Risk, and Protective Factors   391

Lene Symes

> The results of abuse may include repeated abuse, chronic pain, and physical and emotional illnesses. For some, the result is death, but others thrive. Males and females are abused at similar rates, but males are more likely to experience physical assault and females are more likely to experience sexual assault. Males and females experience psychological abuse at the same rates and there is evidence that the effects of psychological abuse are as detrimental to long-term functioning as the effects of physical abuse. This article discusses partner violence in adults and adolescents, child maltreatment, and peer abuse in children and adolescents.

Child Abuse   413

MaryAnn Troiano

> Child abuse can have a long-lasting and devastating effect on the growth and development of infants, children, and adolescents. Studies of abused and neglected children indicate that they have a higher rate of delayed intellectual development, poor school performance, aggressive behaviors, and social and relationship deficits compared with nonmaltreated children. Early recognition and appropriate treatment is one of the most important factors in preventing further child abuse and maltreatment. Every practitioner should be educated on the signs and symptoms of child abuse. The referral to child protective services is a necessity for the future well-being of the child.

**"I know it shouldn't but it still hurts" Bullying and Adults: Implications and
Interventions for Practice**   423

Laura Kelly

> Bullying problems among children and adolescents are well documented but there is scant literature that examines this phenomenon among adults. This article contends that nurses must begin to assess adult patients for this type of violence. Direct questions about being bullied at work or in cyberspace should be added to assessments. Questioning will help bullying victims recognize that what they are going through is not acceptable and not

their fault. It will also help identify patients who may need interventions beyond the treatment of the physically traumatic effects of bullying.

Blind, Deaf, and Dumb: Why Elder Abuse Goes Unidentified   431

Sharon W. Stark

Elder abuse is a growing public health concern that affects elders regardless of residence, socioeconomic status, or geographic locale. Elder abuse includes acts of physical, psychological, verbal, and financial abuses as well as abandonment and neglect. Elder abuse has the potential to occur in multiple settings, whether in the home, rehabilitation centers, long-term care facilities, nursing homes, and/or senior day care centers. Children, family members, friends, and formal caregivers are prospective perpetrators of elder abuse. Public policy changes are necessary to standardize and delineate guidelines and procedures for the detection and prevention of elder abuse in the future.

The Relationship Between Abuse and Depression   437

Kelsey L. Hegarty

Very strong links exist between abuse and depression in clinical practice. Abuse and depression often coexist in the victims and perpetrators of abuse. In nursing practice, responding to patients, particularly women, presenting with depression or depressive symptoms requires an understanding of the underlying and perhaps hidden issues of abuse and violence. Women who have experienced trauma often are diagnosed with depression, when in fact they have symptoms more consistent with posttraumatic stress disorder. Furthermore, depression often improves over time, when women manage to escape the abuse and violence in the relationship.

Family Issues Associated with Military Deployment, Family Violence, and Military Sexual Trauma   445

Cira Fraser

Today's military has a greater percentage of families and children in comparison with previous generations. There are many, and unique, demands on military families made by the ongoing conflicts, and military life can be stressful. The presence of an increasing number of stressors is associated with an increased likelihood of domestic violence in military families and sexual trauma in service members. In this article, literature and research are presented to provide an overview of military deployment and families, and the effect of deployment on families; this is followed by a review of research on family violence and military sexual trauma.

Workplace Violence in Nursing Today   457

Susan Araujo and Laura Sofield

Workplace violence is not a new phenomenon and is often sensationalized by the media when an incident occurs. Verbal abuse is a form of workplace violence that leaves no scars. However, for nurses, the emotional damage to the individual can affect productivity, increase medication errors, incur absenteeism, and decrease morale and overall satisfaction within the nursing profession. This results in staffing turnover and creates a hostile work environment that affects the culture within the organization.

The Impact of Interpersonal Violence on Health Care   465

Rose Knapp

Interpersonal violence is prevalent in our society. Unfortunately, given the current stressors on individuals, families, and communities, the incidences of child abuse, interpersonal violence, and elder abuse are increasing. The economic impact on health care costs is significant. There are many contributing factors to abuse and they are all public health issues that must be addressed for these abuses to cease. This article describes the indicators of interpersonal violence, and outlines strategies for assessment and prevention.

Community Services for Victims of Interpersonal Violence   471

Laura Jannone

Interpersonal violence can be categorized into youth violence, childhood maltreatment, intimate partner violence, elder abuse, or sexual violence. Just as there are several different victims of interpersonal violence, there are various different community services and prevention programs for each particular type of interpersonal violence. This article reviews the literature on community services and prevention available for all victims of interpersonal violence, and examines the literature on whether these programs are effective.

Domestic and Institutional Elder Abuse Legislation   477

Jeanette M. Daly

Statutes pertinent to elder abuse vary widely. This article provides examples of organizational structure, dependency and age of the victim, definitions of abuse, classification of penalties, and investigation processes. Health care providers must learn their state's elder abuse laws and review any operating manuals produced from the statutes or regulations. All health care workers must know and implement the law to protect the welfare of older persons.

Meeting the 2015 Millennium Development Goals with New Interventions for Abused Women   485

Rozina Karmaliani, Shireen Shehzad, Saima Shams Hirani, Nargis Asad, Shela Akbar Ali Hirani, and Judith McFarlane

In a developing country such as Pakistan, where illiteracy, poverty, gender differences, and health issues are prevalent, violence against women is a commonly observed phenomenon. The rising incidences of abuse among women indicate a need to introduce evidence-based community-derived interventions for meeting Millennium Developmental Goals by 2015. This article discusses the application of counseling, economic skills building, and microcredit programs as practical and effective interventions to improve the health outcomes of abused women and, therefore, improving maternal and child health in the Pakistani society.

Index   495

FORTHCOMING ISSUES

March 2012
Tobacco Control
Nancy L. York, PhD, RN, CNE,
Guest Editor

June 2012
Future of Advanced Nursing Practice
Robin Dennison, DNP, MSN, CCNS, RN,
Guest Editor

September 2012
Second Generation Work with QSEN
Joanne Disch, PhD, RN, FAAN, and
Jane H. Barnsteiner, PhD, FAAN,
Guest Editors

December 2012
New Developments in Nursing Education
Mary Ellen Smith Glasgow, PhD, RN,
ACNS-BC, *Guest Editor*

RECENT ISSUES

September 2011
Patient Education
Stephen D. Krau, PhD, RN, CNE,
Guest Editor

June 2011
Culturally Competent Care
Diane B. Monsivais, PhD, CRRN,
Guest Editor

March 2011
**Magnet Environments: Supporting the
Retention and Satisfaction of Nurses**
Karen S. Hill, RN, DNP, NEA-BC, FACHE,
Guest Editor

THE CLINICS ARE NOW AVAILABLE ONLINE!

Access your subscription at:
www.theclinics.com

Preface

Abuse does not emerge by a certain age, happen in a single socioeconomic group, present in a distinct way, or occur in a single setting. Whether in the privacy of one's home or in a public arena such as a daycare or community center or health care facility, infants, children, teenagers, gays, bisexuals, transvestites, elderly, and disabled of all races, cultures, religions, and socioeconomic levels are potential victims of abuse. Abuse can begin innocuously and be sporadic, but usually always escalates over time. Abuse affects individuals, families, communities, and nations. The scope of abuse is enormous. Abuse is not entirely physical. It is emotional, psychological, financial, and/or sexual in nature. Whether one is a victim, witness, or perpetrator of abuse, the health effects are always negative. Some experts believe that exposure to abuse and violence is a contributing factor to chronic disease. Such long-term health consequences have a negative economic impact on society, costing billions of dollars each year.

This issue of *Nursing Clinics of North America* is formatted in chronological order beginning with descriptions of various types of abuse and specific writings about abuse across the lifespan, child abuse, bullying, and elder abuse and their prevalence. The impact of abuse on individuals, families, health care, and society is detailed in writing regarding abuse and depression. An exploration of abuse associated with specialized environments is offered in writings concerning family issues associated with military deployment and workplace violence in nursing. The influence of abuse is elucidated in a writing concerning the impact of interpersonal violence on health care. Finally, innovations designed to address abuse are revealed in writings related to community services for victims of interpersonal violence, domestic, and institutional elder abuse legislation and meeting the United Nations 2015 millennium goals with new interventions for abused women. Overall, education, screening, and responding to abusive situations require the involvement of many at all levels to make changes, develop abuse policies, and support abuse legislation.

Sharon W. Stark, PhD, RN, APN-C, CFN
Monmouth University
Marjorie K. Unterberg School of Nursing and Health Studies
400 Cedar Avenue
West Long Branch, NJ 07764, USA

E-mail address:
swstark@monmouth.edu

Nurs Clin N Am 46 (2011) ix
doi:10.1016/j.cnur.2011.10.001
0029-6465/11/$ – see front matter © 2011 Elsevier Inc. All rights reserved.

Types of Abuse

Janet Mahoney, RN, PhD, APN, ENA-BC

KEYWORDS
- Abuse prevention • Interpersonal violence • Child maltreatment
- Elder abuse • Victim assessment

Let's face it. Abuse should never happen to anyone. All types of abuse are horrific and affect people in all walks of life, regardless of age, educational background, gender, economic status, religion, or nationality. Abuse can harm people physically and emotionally, as well as leave them feeling isolated and lonely. Abuse does not discriminate. It affects children, adults, and older people.

There are many types of abuse. The four most common types of abuse are physical, sexual, emotional, and economic.[1] Abuse is often further categorized into child abuse, intimate partner violence, and elder abuse. Stalking and bullying is considered by some authorities to be types of abuse and are getting more attention in the media.

Some types of abuse are easier to identify than are others. For example, physical abuse is often more identifiable than other types of abuse, although not all types of physical abuse can be seen. Just as serious, and many times more difficult to recognize, are verbal abuse, emotional abuse (psychological abuse), and economic abuse. As with all types of abuse, the signs and symptoms will vary in relation to the frequency and pattern of violence.[2]

CHILD ABUSE

Each year close to 1 million American children are victims of abuse and neglect.[3] Of these young victims, abuse occurred most frequently in children under the age of one. Over half of the abused children were girls, most were white, 21% were Latino, and about 16% were African American.[4]

Data indicates that the incidence of child abuse and neglect is 12 per 1000 children. Four children per day (14,460) children died in 2005 as a result of inflicted trauma. More than 77% of these deaths were children younger than 4 years of age.[4] Although reports of alleged child abuse are not always substantiated during the investigation process, most authorities believe that a large underreporting bias is inherent in the data. There is much more child abuse than is reported.

Child abuse may include signs of abuse and neglect. The Joyful Heart Foundation[5] describes 10 common signs to watch for when child abuse is suspected. Signs and symptoms may include unexplained and unconvincing explanations by parents or

Monmouth University, Marjorie K. Unterberg School of Nursing and Health Studies, 400 Cedar Avenue, West Long Branch, NJ 07764, USA
E-mail address: jmahoney@monmouth.edu

Nurs Clin N Am 46 (2011) 385–390
doi:10.1016/j.cnur.2011.08.005
0029-6465/11/$ – see front matter © 2011 Elsevier Inc. All rights reserved.

care-givers regarding a child's injuries. Abused children may exhibit changes in behavior, such as appearing scared, looking depressed, withdrawing from friends, acting out, or becoming more aggressive. Some children of abuse return to earlier childhood behaviors, such as bedwetting or thumb sucking.[5]

Eating patterns may change and some children may have trouble sleeping. Older abused children may experience changes in school performance and attendance. Abused children may have long absences from school, or may wear clothing inappropriate for the season and climate. Abused children may fear going home after school. Signs of physical abuse include unexplained, repeated, or excessive bruises, broken bones, black eyes, or other injuries. Injuries may be in various stages of healing.[5]

Children who have been sexually abused may not want to tell anyone about the sexual abuse for fear of retaliation from the abuser. Physical signs of sexual abuse may include bruising of the inner thighs, sexually transmitted diseases, and/or pain or itching in the genital area. Children sexually abused by a relative may have been told not to say anything to anyone. For instance, the child may be told that something bad will happen to them or their loved ones if they told anyone about the abuse. The child may have been told that no one will believe his or her stories. These children are vulnerable and live in fear.[5]

Another type of abuse is shaken baby syndrome. Shaken baby syndrome is the leading cause of death seen in abusive head trauma incidents, with an estimated 1200 to 1400 children injured or killed by shaking each year in the United States (US) according the National Center on Shaken Baby Syndrome.[6] Esernio-Jenssen's,[6] 2011 study investigated shaken baby syndrome in 40 infants. He reported that the average age of abused infants was more than 9 months old, with 94% sustaining brain hemorrhage and 82% revealed retinal hemorrhages. Two-thirds (34) of the children were boys and 6 of the 34 died from the injuries. In this study, abusers of shaken baby syndrome ranged in age from 16 to 60 years of age. The female abusers' median age was 34 years. This was significantly higher than the males' median age of 27 years. The investigator stated that, although men were more likely to be seen as perpetrators of shaken baby syndrome, the percentage of female abusers seems to be underestimated.[6]

In this age of ever increasing technology, a new form of violence aimed at children by children has emerged. Electronic aggression is an emerging public health issue. Text messaging allows children to threaten, harass, embarrass, and bully others in Internet chat rooms and on social networking Web sites and Internet blogs. Children can also send aggressive e-mails, pictures, and instant text messages to others via computers, cell phones, and other types of technology. Collectively, this type of behavior is called electronic aggression.[7] The Center for Disease Control (CDC)[7] reports that episodes of victimization are occurring through all forms of technology: 25% in a chat room, 23% on a Web site, 67% with instant messaging, 25% through e-mail, and 16% with text messaging.[7]

Intimate Partner Violence

Intimate partner violence can be defined as the willful intimidation, physical assault, battery, sexual assault, and or other abusive behavior perpetrated by an intimate partner against another.[8] In adults, an estimated 4.8 million women were victims of physical assault by an intimate partner each year.[8] According to the Federal Bureau of Investigation (FBI), more than 3 million women are battered each year. Just as child abuse goes underreported, most cases of intimate partner violence are never reported to the police, and less than one-fifth of victims reporting an injury from intimate partner violence will seek medical treatment following the injury.[9] Ninety-five percent of domestic violence victim are women.[10] Intimate partner violence is a public health problem. Intimate partner violence is violence that occurs between two people in a close relationship. The term "intimate partner" includes current and former spouses and dating partners.[10]

The FBI reported that nearly one-third of all women murdered in the US in 1998 were killed by a current or former intimate partner.[11] Guns were used in almost two-thirds of the homicides. Thirty-seven percent of all women who sought emergency room treatment for violence-related injuries were injured by a current or former spouse, boyfriend, or girlfriend.[11]

Intimate partner violence exists along a continuum from a single episode of violence to ongoing battering. There are four types of violence: physical violence, sexual violence, threats of physical or sexual violence, and emotional abuse. In 2005, 1510 people in the US died at the hands of an intimate partner. The National Violence Against Women survey found that 22.1% of women and 7.4% of men experience physical forms of intimate partner violence at some point in their lives. The cost of intimate partner violence against women, including medical care, mental health services, and lost productivity (eg, time away from work), was an estimated $5.8 billion in 1995.[8]

Intimate violence comes in many forms. Psychological abuse can take the form of constant phone calls, text-messages, e-mails, or instant messages to check up on the abused. This type of abuse is called harassment. The abuser may be extremely jealous of the abused having friends and spending time with other people. The abuser tries to isolate their partner and keep family and friends from interacting with each other. The abuser uses name-calling and puts the person down in front of others or when alone. Abused persons often make excuses for their injuries and may feel like they have to lie about their bruises and injuries. They may feel bad about themselves and be too frightened to speak up for fear of making their partner angry.

The signs for physical abuse include bruises that result from hitting, kicking, punching, grabbing, hair pulling, slapping, biting, and other types of physical harm. Physical abuse is the use of physical force that results in bodily harm, especially in the "bathing suit" zone (abdomen, buttocks, genital area, and upper thighs.[12] Signs and symptoms of physical abuse may include bruises, black eyes, bone fractures, and injuries in various stages of healing. Bruises on the forearms may indicate that victims were trying to defend themselves.[13] The color of bruises may help in establishing a timeline for when the trauma occurred. For instance, 12 to 36 hours after blunt trauma bruises will appear reddish purple, whereas a bruise that occurred a week ago may appear yellowish in a light-skinned person.[13]

Warning signs of intimate partner violence include the abuser being someone who tries to control his or her spouse or significant other's behavior, finances, and social contacts. One of the most telling signs of intimate partner violence is the abused being fearful of his or her spouse or partner. The abused person may be afraid to make the abuser angry in fear of retaliation. The abused may try to cover up bruises and dismiss the abuse as not being a big deal. When a person feels like they have to walk on eggshells to avoid a fight, chances are they are in an abusive relationship. Abusers may lose their temper and break objects at the "drop of a hat" without provocation. Abusers try to isolate their partners by keeping family and friends from interacting with each other.[12]

People of all ages need to be educated about the warning signs of dangerous relationships. Acceptance of violence is a learned behavior. Early intervention for both parties involved in a dating violence situation must be done in a professional and nonjudgmental fashion, always being sensitive to ethic and cultural diversity.[12]

In psychological abuse, the abused person may exhibit low self-esteem. Emotional abuse includes the intentional use of threats, humiliation, intimidation, and isolation.[13] The abuser uses hurting and humiliating remarks as weapons instead of punches and blows. Emotional abuse often starts out very subtly and progresses gradually over time. Emotional abuse is the most difficult type to recognize.[13]

Emotional abuse is characterized by the abuser's manipulation and invalidation of his or her partner. The abuser may refuse to listen or give the silent treatment. Neglect is the most common type of psychological abuse. Abusers cause the abused to lose confidence in themselves to the point that they may question their own perceptions and feelings. Abusers demand having their own way and blame others for their unhappiness, may threaten to end the relationship, totally reject or abandon the abused, give the abused the "cold shoulder," or use other tactics to control the abused.

Elder Abuse

Elder abuse has been one of the last forms of family violence to receive societal attention and is the least reported type of violence. Elder abuse was barely known in the United State until 1978.[14] Nearly 566,000 reports of elder abuse were made nationally in 2003. This is almost 20% more reports than were made in 2000.[15] With the elderly being the fastest growing segment of the US population, the problem of elder abuse is expected to escalate.

According to the Administration on Aging (AOA),[16] there are six types of maltreatment that occur in people over the age of 60 years of age. These include physical abuse, sexual abuse, emotional abuse, neglect, abandonment, and self-neglect.[16]

Elder maltreatment is a significant public health problem. Each year, hundreds of thousands of adults over the age of 60 years are abused, neglected, or financially exploited. The CDC reports that, in the US alone, more than 500,000 older adults are believed abused or neglected each year. These statistics are likely to be an underestimate because many victims are unable or afraid to tell the police, family, or friends about the violence.[17]

Elder abuse can happen to any elder, anywhere. For the elderly, abuse often occurs in the home or in health care facilities. The abuse can be perpetrated by caregivers, strangers, loved ones, or a best friend.[17]

Abuse of the elderly comes in many forms, such as stealing, mismanaging funds, misusing medication, causing psychological distress, withholding food or care, or sexually abusing, exploiting, or confining a person.[18] Signs of elder abuse may include poor hygiene, bedsores, urine odor, repeated infections, dehydration, malnutrition, excoriation or abrasions of the genitalia or the breast area, social isolation, anxiety, and depression. Physical and chemical restraints are forms of abuse.[18]

In financial abuse, the abuser's goal is to control the elder person. Controlling finances can be taken to a point at which an elder does not have access to his or her money or credit cards. The abuser may give the abused a small allowance and expect an account for every penny spent. The abuser may steal from the abused or sabotage the victim's employment by making the victim call out or by calling constantly during working hours. Financial abuse includes withholding basic necessities such as food, clothes, medications, and shelter.[19]

Signs of abuse and neglect in the elderly may include the abused person feeling depressed, anxious, or fearful. The abused person may need to make frequent visits to the emergency room and, more often than not, will give vague explanations about their illness or injuries. Discrepancy in psychosocial and medical history between may point to possible abuse.[19]

Self-neglect occurs when an older person engages in behavior that threatens their own safety, even though they are mentally competent and understand the consequences of their decisions. Symptoms of self-neglect include dehydration, malnutrition, and poor hygiene. The home may be unsanitary or unclean. The person may wear inappropriate or inadequate clothing for the weather and time of year. There may be a lack of medical aids such as eyeglasses, dentures, or hearing aids. The person may choose homelessness.[20]

SUMMARY

Nurses and health care providers play an important role is detecting, assessing, and reporting abuse. Armed with increased knowledge about signs and symptoms of abuse, nurses guide patients to the appropriate resources. Nurses working in the emergency rooms, primary care clinics, and the community should suspect abuse when the injury does not match the story. For example, a patient with injuries to the rib cage may say that they fell off a ladder, when in reality the fractured ribs were caused by being pushed into a staircase. Sometimes, nurses notice mannerisms of the patients. The patients may seem too quiet or say things like "I am such a klutz" or "I don't want to say something that gets him [her] mad." The abused tends to play down the injuries.

Nurses should see red flags go up when a patient's explanation of an injury does not match the injury. Bruises on the body in various stages of healing are a clue for nurses to inquire further and ask questions about a patient's safety. Nurses may say, "I have seen these same bruises on people that are battered" or "Do you feel safe in your home?" Using statements like these can be the impetus for a patient to begin to talk about abuse. Nurses need to be nonjudgmental. It is easy to say, "Why don't you just leave?" In reality, a plan of action for leaving an abusive relationship should be in place whenever someone is thinking of leaving the abuser. Money, shelter, food, and for some people, a change in identity, needs to be thought of in advance.

The goal of abuse prevention is to educate as many people as possible about how to prevent abuse. Nurses must advocate for the vulnerable populations when abuse is suspected. Children, men and women, and the elderly need the help that health care providers can provide. Resources and knowledge are the keys for abolishing abuse. The problem of abuse in children, intimate partners, and elders requires a comprehensive approach that integrates the work of health care, social service, mental health, education, legal, and substance abuse agencies and organizations. There must be collaboration and coordination among all levels of government, private agencies, religious, professional organizations, and volunteers. Health care leaders need to teach patients about abuse and neglect prevention, as well as perform assessment to identify abuse.

REFERENCES

1. Missouri Coalition Against Domestic and Family Violence. Types of abuse 2006. Available at: http://www.mocadsv.org/Resources/CMSResources/pdf/dv101.pdf. Accessed January 26, 2011.
2. A Safe Place.org. What is abuse? Types of abuse 2011. Available at: http://www.asafeplacenh.org/abuse_types.html. Accessed January 26, 2011.
3. Mersch J. Child maltreatment. MedicineNet 2009. Available at: http://www.medicinenet.com/child_abuse/article.htm. Accessed January 26, 2011.
4. US Department of Health and Human Services Administration for Children and Families. Child Maltreatment 2009. Available at: http://www.acf.hhs.gov/programs/cb/pubs/cm09/index.htm. Accessed January 26, 2011.

5. Signs of abuse and neglect in children 2011. Available at: http://www. joyfulheartfoundation.org/childabuse_signsofabuse.htm. Accessed January 26, 2011.
6. Esernio-Jenssen D. In shaken baby syndrome: women as likely to be perpetrators as men 2011. Available at: http://www.nlm.nih.gov.medlineplus/news/fyllstory_109551.html. Accessed January 26, 2011.
7. Hertz MF, David-Ferdon C. Electronic media and youth violence: a CDC issue brief for educators and caregivers. Atlanta (GA): Centers for Disease Control; 2008. Available at: http://www.cdc.gov/Features/dsElectronicAggression. Accessed January 26, 2011.
8. Centers for Disease Control and Prevention. Costs of intimate partner violence against women in the United States 2011; Centers for Disease Control and Prevention: Available at: http://www.cdc.gov/ViolencePrevention/intimatepartner violence/index.html. Accessed January 26, 2011.
9. National Coalition Against Domestic Violence (NCADV). Domestic violence facts. Available at: publicpolicy@ncadv.org. Accessed September 9, 2011.
10. U. S. Department of Justice, Bureau of Justice statistics. Intimate partner violence in the United States 2006. Available at: http://www.cdc.gov/ViolencePrevention/intimatepartnerviolence/index.html. Accessed January 26, 2011.
11. Federal Bureau of Investigation, Uniform Crimes Report. Crime in the United States, 2000. Available at: Publicpolicy@ncadv.org. Accessed January 26, 2011.
12. Ignatavicius D, Workman L. Medical surgical nursing: a nursing process approach. Philadelphia: B. Saunders Company; 2002.
13. Pyrek KM. Forensic nursing. Boca Raton (FL): CRC Press; 2006.
14. Bonnie RJ, Wallace RB. Elder mistreatment: abuse, neglect and exploitation in an aging America. Washington, DC: National Academies Press; 2003.
15. Gearon CJ. State by state elder abuse recourse list 2007. Available at: http://www.arp. org/bulletin/yourlife/statbystate_elder_abuse_resourselist.html. Accessed January 26, 2011.
16. Department of Health and Human Services Administration on Aging. What are the warning signs of elder abuse? 2009. Available at: http://www.aoa.gov/aoaroot/aoa_programs/elder_rights/ea_prevention/whatisea.aspx. Accessed January 26, 2011.
17. Help Guide.org. Elder abuse and neglect. Warning signs, risk factors, prevention and help 2011. Available at: http://www.helpguide.org/mental/elder_abuse_physical_emotional_sexual_neglect.htm. Accessed January 26, 2011.
18. Centers for Disease Control and Prevention. Elder maltreatment prevention 2010. Available at: http://www.cdc.gov/Features/ElderAbuse. Accessed January 26, 2011.
19. Eliopoulos C. Gerontological nursing. 6th edition. Philadelphia: Lippincott Williams & Wilkins; 2005.
20. Hooyman N, Asuman Kiyak H. Social gerontology: a multidisciplinary perspective. 7th edition. Boston: Pearson, Allyn and Bacon; 2005.

Abuse Across the Lifespan: Prevalence, Risk, and Protective Factors

Lene Symes, PhD, RN

KEYWORDS

- Abuse - Interpersonal violence - Intimate partner violence
- Child abuse and neglect

Abuse is "language that condemns or vilifies usually unjustly, intemperately, and angrily" and "physical maltreatment."[1] These definitions do not convey the interpersonal nature of abuse, the conditions in which abuse thrives, or ways to alter those conditions to prevent abuse. They convey nothing about the psychological, physical, and emotional damage that often results from abuse, and they do not suggest a way forward to alleviate the many problems that occur in the aftermath of abuse. This article discusses recent research about those issues related to interpersonal and intimate partner violence (IPV) in adults and adolescents, child maltreatment, and peer abuse in children and adolescents.

The World Health Organization (WHO)[2,3] defines interpersonal violence as: ...violence between family members and intimate partners and violence between acquaintances and strangers that is not intended to further the aims of any formally defined group or cause. Selfdirected violence, war, state-sponsored violence and other collective violence are specifically excluded from these definitions.

Violence includes psychological and emotional ill-treatment, and attempted or actual physical harm, including sexual assault. Forms of violence include child abuse and neglect, IPV, abuse of the elderly, sexual violence, and workplace violence. Although physical and sexual violence are easy to identify, psychological and emotional violence are more difficult to identify.

A search of the PubMed index, limited to nursing journals, humans, and English, indicates nursing's lengthy concern with interpersonal abuse. The first citation about child abuse was in 1973,[4] followed by 2 citations in 1979.[5,6] In 1978, a citation about

---

The author has nothing to disclose.
Texas Woman's University, College of Nursing, 6700 Fannin, Houston, TX 77030, USA
E-mail address: LSymes@twu.edu

0029-6465/11/$ – see front matter © 2011 Elsevier Inc. All rights reserved.

spousal abuse appeared for the first time,[7] followed in 1981 by a citation of an article about battering in pregnancy.[8] In 1983, there was the first citation of an article about elder abuse.[9] The first of the seminal works by Burgess and Holmstrom[10] was cited in 1973. In 1975, their work on assessing trauma following rape was published and included the term rape trauma syndrome.[11] In that article, they describe 2 variations of rape trauma syndrome, compounded reaction and silent reaction, in which the victim has various symptoms but does not talk about the rape. These earlier papers focused primarily on the individual child, woman, or elder who was the primary victim. Later citations include articles with a focus on the infants and children of abused women. For instance, in a 1996 article, McFarlane and colleagues[12] described their findings of the association of abuse during pregnancy with infant birth weight. In a 2010 article, Shay-Zapien and Bullock[13] synthesized the literature examining the impact of abuse on women, fetuses, and children. This brief and ad hoc trajectory suggests an increasing awareness of the complex issues related to abuse.

WHO ARE THE VICTIMS OF ABUSE?

To effectively assess for abuse, nurses need to understand the risk factors for abuse (**Tables 1–3**). Victims of abuse include women, men, adolescents, the unborn, infants, and children. Society as a whole is a victim, given the costs of health care and of lost productivity secondary to IPV, and, in the case of homicide, the loss of lifetime contributions. Abuse is most likely to occur when there is inequality, whether social, political, physical, or financial. Gender inequality may lead to ongoing abuse when victims do not seek help. Mongolian women who are abused and accept gender inequality may keep silent because they value respect for the authority of husbands and because they consider the abuse to be shameful.[14]

To establish meaningful social policies for prevention and treatment of abuse, it is important to understand the prevalence and risk factors for abuse, as well as the costs related to abuse. There are barriers to establishing accurate prevalence and risk data, and to understanding all the costs associated with abuse. Problems include the use of different definitions by different researchers, policy makers, and clinicians, as well as bias in determining abuse, and limitations on self-report data. There is evidence that the prevalence of abuse is usually underreported. The issues are complex and the full extent of the loss of physical, emotional, and psychological function may only become apparent with time, and problems may be transmitted from generation to generation. Current research findings about the prevalence of, risk factors for, and protective factors against, various forms of abuse are described later.

International Prevalence Studies

Garcia-Moreno and colleagues.[15] used data collected from ever-partnered women, aged 15 to 49 years, in 10 countries (n = 24,097), from 2000 to 2003, for the World Health Organization (WHO) Multi-Country Study on Women's Health and Domestic Violence, to evaluate the lifetime prevalence of physical and sexual partner violence. They found that the prevalence varied from 15% in Japan city (n = 1277) to 71% in Ethiopia province (n = 2261). In the United States, findings from a survey (n>70,156), conducted in 18 states and territories, were that approximately 1 in 4 women had been victims of some form of lifetime IPV.[16] In a secondary analysis of survey data collected in 19 countries, from 2% (Australia, Cambodia, Denmark, Philippines) to 13.5% (Uganda) of pregnant women experienced IPV.[17] Given findings from a prospective study of pregnant women in the United States (n = 691), where 1 in 6 women (16%) were found to experience physical violence during pregnancy,[18] it is

Table 1
If the male partner has these, or if she has these, a woman is more likely to be abused

Risk Factors for Female Abuse	Male Partner	Female Partner
Alcohol abuse	Yes	Yes
Young age	Not reported	Yes
Cohabitation (not married)	Yes	Yes
Childhood abuse (physical or sexual)	Yes	Yes
Emotion dysregulation	Not reported	Yes
Partner's mother was abused	Yes	Yes
Perpetration of violence as an adult	Yes	Yes
Children from previous relationship	Not reported	Yes
Long-term physical or mental condition	Yes	Yes
Low education (note: both partners having high school education is a protective factor)	Yes	Yes
Unskilled worker	Yes	Not reported
5 or more living in 1 home	Yes	Yes
Low socioeconomic status of family	Yes	Yes
Misperceives woman as sexually interested	Yes	N/A
Accepts gender inequality	Yes	Yes
Finds actions justifiable	Yes	Yes
Believes that IPV is a private matter or shameful	Not reported	Yes
Witnessed threats of, or actual, interparental violence	—	Yes
Woman working in traditional male occupation (such as military)	N/A	Yes

Table 2
If the male partner has these, he is more likely to be abused, and if a woman has these, she is more likely to abuse her male partner

Risk Factors for Male Abuse	Male Partner	Female Partner
Greater than 5 alcoholic drinks per day	Yes	Yes
Drug use	Yes	Yes
Delinquent behavior	Yes	Yes
History of childhood sexual assault	Yes	—

Table 3
The child with these family or caregiver factors, or who has some of these factors, is more likely to be abused

Risk Factors (See Ref.[42])	Child Abuse	Child Neglect
Unrelated man present in home	Yes	—
Parental separations of greater than 1 mo	—	Yes
Disorganized/chaotic family	—	Yes
Lack of marital harmony and father involvement (harsh discipline/lack of warmth or engagement with child)	Yes	Yes
Lack of parental supervision	—	Yes
Caregiver/parent has initial difficult bonding with infant	Yes	Yes
Caregiver/parent does not understand child development/ unrealistic expectations	Yes	—
Caregiver/parent approves of physical punishment, poor parenting skills	Yes	Yes
Family is socially isolated	Yes	Yes
Caregiver/parent misuses alcohol or drugs	Yes	Yes
Physical, developmental, or mental health problems of family member(s)	Yes	Yes
High levels of unemployment, poor housing, lack of services in community	Yes	Yes
Child has high needs or a more affectively expressive style (vs interpersonal reserve, self-confidence, and self-reliance)	Yes	Yes

likely that the results of Devries and colleagues[17] underestimate the prevalence of abuse during pregnancy.

Abramsky and colleagues,[19] like Garcia-Moreno and colleagues,[15] also used data from the WHO Multi-Country Study on Women's Health and Domestic Violence. They studied factors linked with IPV occurring in the 12 months before data collection, in ever-partnered women aged 15 to 49 years (n = 19,519). They found that alcohol abuse by either or both partners, cohabitation, young age of women, either partner experiencing childhood abuse in the form of beating for the male or sexual assault for the female, a history of either or both partners' mothers being abused, and either partner experiencing or perpetrating other forms of violence in adulthood increased IPV risk for women. Being in a formal marriage in which both partners have secondary education decreased the IPV risk. Women who had children from previous relationships were at greater risk compared with other women. At first, high socioeconomic status seemed to protect against IPV, but this was less apparent after the researchers adjusted for confounding or mediating variables. Li and colleagues,[20] in a study of low-income pregnant women in Jefferson County, Alabama, also found that being unmarried and alcohol use were associated with increased risk for IPV.

Daigneault and colleagues[21] found that women who had a history of childhood sexual assault were from 2 to 5 times more likely than other women to experience adult physical, psychological, and sexual IPV with their current partner (odds ratio = 2.4, 2.9, and 4.8 respectively), after controlling for numerous factors including income level, marital status, and alcohol use. They also found that women with limitations caused by a long-term physical or mental condition were more likely than other women to experience psychological, physical, or sexual IPV (odds ratio = 1.73, 1.67, and 2.62) with their current partner.

Ali and colleagues[22] conducted a study to evaluate the prevalence, frequency, and risk factors for IPV victimization among women (n = 759 married women, 25–60 years old) in Pakistan. Women reported past-year and lifetime rates of physical violence (56.3% and 57.6% respectively), sexual violence (53.4%, 54.5%), and psychological abuse (81.8%, 83.6%). Risk factors varied by type of violence. For physical violence, the main risk factors were the husband's low educational attainment, unskilled worker status, and having 5 or more family members living in 1 household. For sexual violence, the main risk factors were the woman's low educational attainment, the low socioeconomic status of the family, and 5 or more family members living in 1 household. For psychological violence, the risk factors were the husband being an unskilled worker and the low socioeconomic status of the family. The investigators concluded that repeated violence by husband against wife is treated with indifference because of the prevailing attitude that IPV is a private matter and that the actions are justifiable. This study is noteworthy for the careful training of midwives who collected the data and the random sampling used to select study participants. The investigators noted that the prevalence that they found is similar to the prevalence reported for Iran and higher than those for Vietnam, India, and Bangladesh. They suggested that the high prevalence for IPV against women revealed by this study is explained by the gender inequality accepted in Pakistan and by the trust the participants had in the midwives who collected the data.

Risk Factors for Abuse

Using data collected from 393 families in Baltimore, Maryland, O'Campo and colleagues[23] found that more families from the lowest (income<51% of poverty level) and highest (>335% of poverty level) income groups reported higher rates of IPV (58.6% and 61.4% of families, respectively) compared with families from the middle groups, in which families with incomes of 50% to 99%, 100% to 199%, and 200% to 334% of the poverty level were less likely to report IPV (45.9%, 41.2%, and 47.1% respectively).

Rennison and Planty[24] questioned research findings of racial disparities in IPV rates in the United States. To evaluate the issue, they applied 3 steps to analyzing data from approximately 336,295 households and 641,750 individuals, collected from 1993 to 1999 for the National Crime Victimization Survey (NCVS). In the first step, where IPV was grouped by race, overall rates of IPV were greater for black people (6.7 per 1000) versus white people (4.6 per 1000). In the second step, where gender was controlled for, IPV rates were greater for black women (10.7 per 1000) than white women (7.8 per 1000). In the third step, where race was controlled for, there were no significant differences between racial groups for IPV. White women with household annual incomes less than $7500 had 20.3 IPV experiences per 1000, whereas black women had 21.0.

According to the 2004 WHO report, *Effects of Economic Factors and Policies on Interpersonal Violence*, most studies of economic inequality and violence focused on homicide.[3] Although not well studied, it may be that it is income inequality, rather than income level alone, that is related to IPV.

Cicchetti,[25] from the Institute of Child Development at the University of Minnesota, described existing research on psychological and biological determinants of resilience in maltreated children. In abused children, these factors may protect them from future abuse and from other untoward outcomes. Having ego control (being able to monitor and control impulses) and ego resiliency (flexibility in managing affect and behavior for a given situation) were protective, whereas, having less ego control, and thus being more affectively expressive, resulted in poorer outcomes. Those who are more affectively expressive may draw attention to themselves, resulting in a greater risk for maltreatment.

Sexual Abuse: Gender Differences and Risk Factors

Young and colleagues[26] emphasize that how sexual assault is measured greatly influences the estimates of prevalence. More specific measures that include multiple questions about a variety of sexual behaviors and a variety of methods of coercion result in higher prevalence rates for sexual assault. Using a tool that measured petting, kissing, and intercourse, and the methods of verbal pressure, use of authority, and violence, to evaluate sexual victimization in 1086 7th to 12th graders, they found that peer sexual assault (being kissed, hugged, sexually touched, or made to do something else sexual) rates were 26% for boys and 51% for girls. Of the female high school students who reported sexual assault, 6% reported forced oral sex, 12% rape, and 1% attempted rape. Of the male high school students, 3% reported rape. These results make clear the importance of defining what is measured. It is also important to consider the context in which the surveys are conducted. Those seeking health care may have a higher prevalence of abuse. Of girls and women, aged 14 to 20 years attending a health clinic in the eastern United States (n = 356), 45% reported physical or sexual abuse by a dating partner.[27]

Childhood abuse increases the risk of adolescent and adult victimization, directly, and indirectly. Men who report childhood sexual assault, compared with other men, are more likely to experience psychological (odds ratio = 1.9) and physical abuse (odds ratio = 3.0) by their intimate partner. Men with physical or mental limitations who had experienced childhood physical assault were at higher risk for IPV. Having a partner who drank alcohol to excess also increased the men's risk of IPV.[21] Data from a nationally representative, US longitudinal study indicated that adolescent boys (n = 1806, 12–17 years old) who engaged in high-risk behaviors (> 5 alcoholic drinks in any day or alcohol intoxication, drug use, or delinquent behavior) were significantly more likely than others to have a past history of abuse and were at higher risk for future victimization. Adolescent girls (n = 1808) in the same study who had a history of sexual abuse were at higher risk than other girls for future victimization and for engaging in future high-risk behavior, and future high-risk behavior was significantly associated with future sexual abuse.[28]

After controlling for physical, psychological, and neglect abuse, childhood sexual assault was the best predictor of adult sexual risk behaviors (unprotected sex and more lifetime sexual partners) among women (n = 414) who attended a publicly funded clinic for treating sexually transmitted diseases located in the United States.[29] Among 752 US college women, 6.3% reported childhood sexual assault, 25.5% reported childhood physical assault, and 17.8% reported rape during adolescence and/or adulthood. There was a significant relationship between both childhood physical and sexual assault and adolescent/adult rape. Of those with a history of child-hood sexual assault, 29.8% experienced adolescent/adult rape and, of those with a history of childhood physical assault, 24.3% experienced adolescent/adult rape. A history of any of the 3 forms of abuse was associated with higher levels of emotion dysregulation (difficulty identifying and regulating emotional states, lower levels of emotional acceptance, and increased experiential avoidance). A path analysis showed that those with childhood physical and/or sexual assault were at greater risk for emotion dysregulation and risky sex, and both emotion dysregulation and risky sex increased the risk for adult rape. Direct paths between child maltreatment and rape were not significant and were not included in the final model.[30] In contrast, Walsh and colleagues[31] found childhood sexual assault to be the strongest independent predictor of forced adult sexual assault. McKinney and colleagues[32] found that, among US men (1615 couples) who had experienced moderate physical abuse as a child, the odds ratio of perpetrating IPV was 3.9. For those who experienced severe physical abuse, the odds ratio of perpetrating IPV was 4.5. Women were at increased risk for victimization if they had witnessed interparental threats of violence (odds ratio 1.9) or actual violence (odds ratio 3.4) as a child.

There is some evidence that men and women differ in their perception of the sexual interest of others, and that sexually coercive men are more likely to misperceive tar-geted women as sexually interested. Little is known about the basis for the mispercep-tions. Some have suggested that the basis is evolutionary, whereas others suggest that they are related to social processes or individual learning. Further research by cognitive scientists is needed to develop an understanding of the processes that underpin the misperceptions and then to develop effective intervention strategies.[33]

Women who work in traditionally male occupations in which workers and super-visors are primarily male are at greater risk for sexual harassment. Vogt and colleagues,[34] in a study using data from 2037 former reservists, found that attitudes toward women are associated with several military characteristics that predict toler-ance for sexual harassment. Individuals who witnessed threatened or actual interpar-ental IPV during childhood are more likely to perpetrate IPV or be victimized.

There is evidence that men and women experience significantly different types of IPV, with women being more likely to report injury and sexual assault. Brieding and colleagues[16] found that 1 in 7 men reported being victims of some form of lifetime IPV. This finding suggests that US men experience lifetime IPV a little more than half as often as women, differing from the male IPV prevalence reported by others. The men in the study were significantly less likely to report IPV-related injury compared with women. In contrast, in a Canadian study, men (n = 7823) and women (n = 9170), with a current or previous partner, had significantly different, but much closer, rates of physical IPV: 7% for men versus 8.5% for women. Differences in rates of psycholog-ical IPV were not statistically significant: 18.8% for men and 19.2% for women. Results from the same study suggest that Canadian men are not significantly more likely to have experienced childhood physical assault (3.1%) than women (2.8%), whereas Canadian women are much more likely to have experienced childhood sexual assault (7.9%) than men (1.9%) and significantly more likely to have experienced adult sexual IPV (1.7% vs 0.2%).[21] Findings from a study of 705 adult men living in Virginia were that 12.9% had experienced lifetime sexual assault. The investigators stated that sexual assault of men is underreported.[35]

Abuse During Pregnancy and Subsequent Health Outcomes

Three recently published studies on 3 continents (Europe and North and South Amer-ica) found that women who experience IPV during or following their pregnancies are at increased risk for postpartum depression. In Italy, 292 women were interviewed while hospitalized following birth and again 8 months later. At the second interview, 10% of the participants reported postpartum violence from a partner or other family member, and 5% had high psychological distress. For women who reported violence, the odds ratio for depressive symptoms was 19.17.[36] In the United States, researchers used data from the Kentucky Women's Health Registry (n = 5380, 2508 with history of IPV) to assess the association between past IPV exposure and postpartum depression. Adult physical and stalking IPV exposure were each associated with postpartum depression (adjusted odds ratio 1.48 and 1.39, respectively). Each additional type of IPV experienced added to the strength of the association.[37] Researchers[38] investigated the association of psychological, physical, and sexual violence during pregnancy with postpartum depression in Brazilian women. Of 1045 women, 270 (25.8%) had postpartum depression and 28% of all the women reported experiencing psychological violence by their partner. More frequent psychological violence was more strongly associated with postpartum depression. The adjusted odds ratios were 1.73 for those experiencing 1 or 2 episodes, 2.72 for those experiencing 3 or 4 episodes, and 3.79 for those experiencing 5 or more episodes of emotional violence. After adjusting for emotional violence, the adjusted odds ratio for physical or sexual violence was not significant, highlighting the effect of psychological abuse.

Maternal IPV physical victimization is associated with infant (<12 months) and child (12 months to <60 months) death and morbidity. Using data from the 2005 to 2006 National Family Health Survey of India, Ackerson and Subramanian[39] found that maternal physical IPV was associated with child death, independently of the child's gender (infant risk ratio 1.21; child risk ratio 1.24). Associations with sexual and psychological IPV were not as strong. It is not known whether the deaths resulted from mothers' inability to care for their children or whether the children experienced direct physical violence. Rico and colleagues[40] evaluated maternal exposure to IPV and maternal IPV victimization and child nutrition and mortality using data collected in surveys in Egypt, Honduras, Kenya, Malawi, and Rwanda. They found that the prevalence of maternal exposure to IPV (since 15 years of age) ranged from 15.5% in Honduras to 46.2% in Kenya. In Kenya, Malawi, and Honduras, maternal exposure to IPV was associated with higher mortality in children less than 2 years old, with the highest association (odds ratio 1.42) in Kenya. Silverman and colleagues[41] used survey data collected in 2004 in Bangladesh to evaluate the association between maternal IPV experiences and morbidity (acute respiratory infection and diarrhea within the past 2 weeks) in children less than 6 years old. They found that 42% of the mothers had experienced IPV from their husbands in the prior year. Mothers who had experience IPV were more likely to report that their children had recent acute respiratory infections (adjusted odds ratio 1.37) and diarrhea (adjusted odds ratio 1.65). The prevalence of IPV was determined from questions asked of the fathers/husbands, not of the mothers/wives. Information about the children's health status came from the mothers.

Child Abuse and Risk Factors

The true extent of childhood maltreatment is not known[42] and estimates are that from one-half to four-fifths of child-maltreatment cases are not known to child protective services. Self-reports of child maltreatment may not be inclusive because of the age when the maltreatment occurred, the type of abuse, or the individual's sense of having deserved punishment. Official reports are likely to be subject to bias, resulting in overreporting or underreporting.

In a study exploring the extent to which school, police, and medical authorities know about child and adolescent experiences of violence, abuse, and crime victimizations, Finkelhor and colleagues[43] interviewed parents of children (n = 4549) aged 0 to 9 years, and children aged 10 to 17 years, about child or adolescent abuse experiences and whether the abuse experiences were known to the authorities. They found that 58.3% of the children and adolescents had at least 1 direct victimization, not including witnessing domestic assault during the prior year. For 45.7% of those who had experienced direct victimization, some authority knew of at least 1 of their experiences. The victimizations known to authorities were typically more severe, such as sexual abuse by a known adult (69/0%) or unknown adult (76.1%), kidnapping (73.5%), and gang or group assault (70.1%). Least known to the authorities were peer and sibling assault (16.9%), dating violence (15.2%), completed and attempted rape (14%), and statutory rape (3.4%). The investigators compared the results with an earlier study that used data from 1992, and concluded that there is some evidence that disclosure to authorities has increased with time.

Childhood neglect may be more difficult to measure than childhood sexual and physical assault, given that it is often the absence rather than the presence of behavior. Maughan and Moore[44] discussed variations in how child neglect has been defined. They provided examples of differences in meaning applied by researchers compared with clinicians. They reported that some researchers limit definitions of neglect to parent-child interactions, independent of current and future negative effects, whereas others include community and child deficits, also without considering long-term outcomes. In contrast, clinicians are interested in neglect because of the link with current and long-term outcomes. They used a well-established longitudinal data set to look for the associations between neglect and future delinquency. Rather than using data from children on child protection registries, the investigators evaluated a data set drawn from the community-based Cambridge Study in Delinquent Development (n = 411 males, living in London, UK). The initial data were collected in 1961 and 1962 when the children were 8 or 9 years old. Additional data were collected up to 6 times, the last being when the participants were 24 years. Data sources included the children, their parents, their teachers, their peers, and the Central Criminal Record Office in London. Adult delinquency included serious or criminal offenses such as theft, burglary, and the unauthorized taking of a motor vehicle. Thirty-nine parenting behavior variables were evaluated using factor analysis and the 4 retained factors were then evaluated using logistic regression to compare the 4 factors with the presence of adult delinquency after controlling for poverty, age, ethnic origin, socioeconomic status, and verbal intelligence quotient (IQ). The 4 factors were parental separations (>1 month separation from a natural or operative parent), disorganized/chaotic home (family size, overcrowding, care of interior of home, noticeable neglect of child's clothing, hygiene, or food), marital harmony and father's involvement (attitude of father as warm, passive, neglecting, or cruel; discipline of father; disagreement or inconsistency between parents; dominance of parents), and parental supervision (trips, sports, movies, clubs, friends' homes). Of the 4 factors, they found that 2 (disorganized/chaotic, parental supervision) were significantly associated with adult delinquency.

Peer victimization among youth has multiple forms. Turner and colleagues[45] evaluated data collected using a nationally representative sample of US children and adolescents (n = 2999 children, 55% non-Hispanic white, 20% non-Hispanic black, 5% other, and 19% Hispanic; 49.5% boys and 50.5% girls), from 6 to 17 years old (31% 6–9 years old, 31% 10–13 years old, 39% 14–17 years old). Data were collected during telephone interviews. If the child was less than 10 years old, the main caregiver was interviewed. For those more than 10 years old, a short interview was conducted with the adult caregiver and the main interview with the child or adolescent. Findings included that more than 22% had experienced at least 1 type of peer physical assault (boys 28.6%, girls 15.3%), 5% had experienced physical intimidation, 20% had experienced emotional victimization, 6.6% had experienced sexual victimization (boys 4.8%, girls 8.5%), 14.5% experienced property crime, and 2.7% experienced Internet harassment. Of peer assaults, 41.5% occurred at locations not related to school, but 78% of bias attacks (being hit or attacked for skin color, religion, nationality, physical disability, or sexual orientation) occurred in school.

PREVALENCE OF PARENTAL VIOLENCE AND CONSEQUENCES FOR YOUNGSTERS

Knutsen and colleagues[46] describe the difficulties of obtaining accurate prevalence rates for children's exposure to parental IPV. Areas of major difficulty include obtaining data from fathers and cohabiting men, and that the child may have had sequential exposure to multiple adult partners of the mother. Law enforcement records, when available, are unlikely to include data about the circumstances of a child's exposure to parental IPV. Few studies of children's exposure to parental IPV have controlled for socioeconomic status (household poverty, economically disadvantaged neighborhoods, community violence). The investigators conducted secondary analysis studies. They reviewed data from samples of economically disadvantaged mothers with children aged from 4 to 8 years, living in rural north central Wisconsin (n = 100 mothers) or in small urban and suburban communities in southeastern Iowa (n = 102 mothers). Among their findings were that physical violence between the mothers and their current adult partners occurred in almost 20% of the Iowa sample and almost 35% of the Wisconsin sample. There was no association between mother's reports of violence with current partners and violence with past partners. When current and prior relationships were considered, from 35% to 40% of the children were, at some time, reared in a household with adult physical IPV. In their discussion, they cite evidence that children are at greater risk for maltreatment and injury when an unrelated man is present, but raise the possibility that a man in the household may provide buffering against the effects of poverty on the child and, if positive, may buffer against outcomes of previous exposure to IPV. They note that parenting may mediate the effect of IPV on child psychosocial adjustment, with children who feel parental support being buffered from adverse consequences of parental IPV. In a prospective study of risk factors for child maltreatment, families of 224 children were recruited from urban pediatric primary care clinics. At entry into the study, none of the children had a child protective services (CPS) report. The children were followed for 10 years, to approximately12 years old. At the conclusion of the study, 97 (43%) children had a CPS report. The investigators found 5 risk factors that predicted CPS reports: child's low performance on a standardized developmental assessment, mother having less than a high school education, maternal drug use, maternal depressive symptoms, and more than 1 child in the family (with each additional child adding to the risk).[47] The mothers were not assessed for posttraumatic stress disorder (PTSD).

Children who witness IPV are at risk for mental health problems.[48] Of 140 children screened for PTSD after their families sought services at a women's center and shelter, 124 had at least 5 symptoms of PTSD related to IPV. Although Cohen and colleagues[48] write that some mothers rightfully view ensuring safety, housing, and other necessities as higher priorities than mental health treatment of their children, in the context of their circumstances (facing multiple traumas during therapy, possible homelessness, repeated IPV, and legal and financial difficulties), they also found evidence that, when mothers and children (aged 7 to 14 years) received mental health treatment in the form of 8 sessions of cognitive behavioral therapy, there was a decrease in serious adverse risks (serious physical IPV, reportable episodes of child abuse, child self-injury, and problems requiring psychiatric hospitalization) to the children. Among children in their sample receiving the usual community treatment (n = 32) of 8 weeks of child-centered therapy, 10 (31%) experienced serious adverse risks, whereas, in the group receiving community-provided trauma-focused cognitive behavioral therapy (n = 43), only 2 (5%) experienced serious adverse risks (z = 2.9, P<.005). This discrepancy shows the importance of evidence-based interventions for mothers and their children. The rate of serious adverse effects among children in similar circumstances, but without any intervention, is not addressed.

Children who witness IPV are also at risk for physical health problems. Brieding and Ziembroski[49] found significantly higher asthma rates among children of women who had experienced lifetime IPV (18.7%) compared with children of women who had not experienced lifetime IPV (14.4%). No significant difference was found for children of men who had or had not experienced IPV. The researchers controlled for other variables significantly associated with children's asthma. Their results were from the population-based data set collected in 2005 from 10 US states/territories in the Behavioral Risk Factor Surveillance System (BRFSS) survey.

In the study by Turner and colleagues[45] of US children and adolescents from 6 to 17 years old (31% 6–9 years, 31% 10–13 years, 39% 14–17 years), with demographic variables held constant, each category of peer victimization was significantly associated with trauma symptoms, from physical intimidation (β = 0.13, P<.001) to emotional victimization (β = 0.28, P<.001). Although all the forms of peer victimization had significant independent effects on trauma symptoms, experiencing multiple forms of peer victimization had the strongest association with trauma symptoms (β = 0.38, P<.001). Two forms of victimization not always included in bullying research, peer sexual victimization (β = 0.20, P<.001) and peer-perpetrated property crime (β = 0.25, P<.001), were associated with trauma symptoms. The investigators suggested that the criterion that bullying occurs in situations of unequal power needs to be further analyzed and argue that "violence, aggression, harassment and denigration are wrong and harmful, however often and in whatever context they occur."

In Holland, researchers compared a control group of adult individuals with no childhood abuse (n = 97, 33% men, 67% women) with individuals who reported childhood emotional abuse before age 16 years (n = 84, 34.5% men, 65.5% women). Current mental health diagnoses were determined for major depressive disorder, anxiety disorder, comorbid major depression and anxiety disorders, and no mental health symptoms (the healthy control group). All were unmedicated. Those with childhood emotional abuse were significantly (P = .01) more likely to have comorbid major depressive disorder and anxiety disorder (30 of 84), compared with those without childhood emotional abuse (13 of 97). Those with no mental health diagnoses were significantly less likely to report childhood emotional maltreatment (40 of 97 vs 13 of 84). Specialized magnetic resonance imaging techniques were used to evaluate for neuroanatomic correlates of childhood emotional abuse. Findings were that, independently of mental health diagnostic status and gender, having self-reported childhood emotional abuse was associated with a significant reduction in predominantly left dorsal medial prefrontal cortex volume. The researchers concluded that this finding may help with understanding the increased emotional sensitivity in those with childhood emotional abuse.[50] These findings suggest an explanation for the usefulness of cognitive behavioral therapy (CBT) for victims of trauma. CBT provides strategies that help individuals modulate emotional responses and thus may help those with increased emotional sensitivity to function with less emotional reactivity.

OUTCOMES OF ABUSE BEYOND THE IMMEDIATE TRAUMA

"In virtually all cases and for all reasons, acceptance of wife-beating was higher among women who had experienced abuse than among those who had not."[51(p10)]

Much of the research discussed in this article makes clear the destructive impact of emotional IPV, which may be easier to overlook than physical and sexual IPV. Not discussed are the secondary outcomes of IPV. For example, the parenting difficulties related to having major depression or anxiety symptoms, and their impact on the functioning of the initial victims' children. IPV victimization may lead to chronic pain and psychological and physical illnesses. Much of the research on outcomes has focused on women and children victims of IPV. When men who have been victims of IPV are included in outcome studies, the results are similar. For example, Wilson and Widom[52] found that adults, men or women, who had documented child abuse (physical or sexual abuse, or neglect, ages 0 to 11 years) were at higher risk for sexually risky behaviors in middle adulthood (approximately 41 years).

Women who have experienced interpersonal violence (IPV) are more likely than women without such experiences to suffer from chronic pain and other physical and psychological illnesses. Bonomi and colleagues[53] completed a telephone survey of women who were members of a large US health plan to determine their abuse status. Data from the women's health insurance records were retrieved and a comparison of women reporting abuse in the past year (n = 242) versus never-abused women (n = 1686) was conducted. After adjusting for age, women reporting abuse had a greater relative risk for psychological/mental problems, musculoskeletal problems, female reproductive disorders, acute respiratory tract infections, gastro-esophageal reflux disease, chest pain, abdominal pain, urinary tract infections, headaches, contusions, abrasions, and lacerations. In a community of 292 women (average of 20 months after separation from abuser) more than one-third experienced disabling pain (measured by the Von Korff Chronic Pain Grade) long after leaving the abusive partners and after controlling for numerous factors. Women with disabling pain were more likely to have histories of child abuse, adult sexual assault, more severe spousal abuse, lifetime abuse-related injuries, symptoms of depression and PTSD, lifetime suicide attempts, difficulty sleeping, and unemployment. In addition, they had more visits to a family doctor and psychiatrist and used more medication than was prescribed. More interference with daily life was attributed to swollen/painful joints (43.2%) than to back, head, stomach, pelvic, or bowel pain.[54] These 2 studies support the findings from numerous earlier studies that women with a history of IPV have a higher risk of chronic pain and other physical and mental health problems compared with women without IPV history. Neither report included information about whether the women had children. However, it is clear that there are situational, emotional, and physical outcomes associated with IPV, which may influence the children of women with IPV history, directly or indirectly.

PTSD and depression are common to those with a history of abuse, either individually or as comorbid conditions. Taft and colleagues[55] evaluated factors associated with PTSD-depression comorbidity in adult women survivors of rape or assault with symptoms of PTSD (n = 162). All participants met diagnostic criteria for PTSD and slightly more than half (52%) met diagnostic criteria for comorbid depression. They found that PTSD-only participants reported higher childhood sexual abuse levels than those with comorbid PTSD and depression, and the group with both reported more distorted trauma-related beliefs, dissociation, PTSD severity, and depression severity. The investigators concluded that PTSD and depression comorbidity do not seem to be a function of symptom overlap.

Mental Health Consequences of Abuse

There is increasing evidence that chronic pain and other physical problems resulting from IPV are mediated by symptoms of PTSD and, to a lesser degree, depression. Woods and collaborators[56] showed that PTSD symptoms mediate the association between IPV and a proinflammatory cytokine, thus indicating a likely pathway, via the hypothalamus-pituitary-adrenal (HPA) axis, from IPV to increased pain and physical symptoms. Wuest and colleagues[57] considered abuse-related injury and PTSD symptom severity as mediators between 3 categories of IPV (assaultive IPV severity, psychological IPV severity, and child abuse severity) and chronic pain. They found that both PTSD symptom severity and abuse-related injury were significant mediators of assaultive IPV severity (β = 0.06 and 0.06, respectively) and child abuse severity (β = 0.13 and 0.05, respectively) with pain, but not of psychological abuse with pain. Child abuse severity made the greatest contribution to the model (β = 0.35). Assaultive IPV severity (β = 0.12) had significant indirect effects on pain. Psychological IPV had only direct effects on the model (β = 0.20). The model they tested accounted for almost 38% of the variance in pain. In a second data analysis, they added depressive symptoms to the model, and increasing the variance in pain accounted for slightly more than 40%. Not only does this study help explain possible pathways to chronic pain but it also highlights the importance of developing interventions to prevent child abuse.

Like the Dutch study of neuroanatomy, another study also suggests that trauma results in physiologic changes that are independent of mental health symptoms. Tucker and colleagues[58] evaluated symptoms of PTSD and depression and assessed autonomic reactivity by comparing the blood pressure and pulse of 60 survivors of the 1995 Oklahoma City bombing with those of 60 community members matched for gender and age. They found that PTSD, but not depression, symptoms were more common among the survivors, even though they did not reach clinically relevant levels. They include a figure in their manuscript that illustrates their findings that the survivors had significantly higher resting heart rates than the comparison group. After resting, all subjects participated in a semistructured interview designed to elicit memories of the bombing event. Although all the participants had significant increases in autonomic measures, survivors had significantly larger responses than those in the comparison group during the interview. Although the comparison group returned to baseline on the postinterview assessment, survivors maintained significant increases in autonomic response. There was not a significant association between PTSD symptoms and autonomic measures. The investigators noted that the greater physiologic reactivity of the survivor group is consistent with findings from physiologic assessment studies of chronic PTSD, but the survivors in this group did not have clinically evident levels of PTSD. They discussed literature by other researchers with similar findings for hostage survivors. They raised the possibility that the physiologic response is adaptive, possibly facilitating effective actions in future disasters.

Another possibility is that the physiologic response is not only adaptive, aiding response to future stresses, but is also maladaptive, leading to the increased pain and chronic illness noted in survivors of IPV. There is considerable research evaluating the theory that the HPA axis is dysregulated in survivors of trauma and that the dysregulation leads to a chronic inflammatory state and results in the high levels of chronic disease, including cardiovascular disease, noted in survivors of IPV.[56]

What should be Considered when Assessing for Abuse?

Health care providers may wonder whether it is helpful to ask someone whether they have experienced IPV or rape. In an early effort to address this issue, Clements and Ogle[59] compared college women who acknowledged IPV or rape with those who did not in response to a direct question about their IPV or rape history. They then had the women complete 2 scales designed to measure IPV and sexual assault history. Women were classified into 2 groups: those whose responses were consistent across measures and those whose response to the direct question differed from the experiences they identified on the scales. Particularly in the rape groups, those who did not acknowledge the rape on the direct question reported greater disability, impaired coping, and greater psychological distress than controls and other groups. This finding raises questions about how best to ask about abuse issues. Simply asking someone whether they have been abused is not enough. Having time to ask about specific types of events with empathy and a coherent plan for follow-up is important. Further study is needed to learn whether acknowledging will help those individuals who do not acknowledge. It may be that there is a difference between the 2 groups beyond the differences in acknowledging rape experience.

It may be difficult for nurses who have their own IPV experiences to ask others about IPV. Nurses may be concerned that they will offend their patient if they ask about personal safety. They may be uncertain about how to bring up the issue, what is important, and what to do with the information. In addition, it may seem secondary to the work at hand and of lesser priority than other issues. Two recent articles emphasize the need for training to prepare nurses for this work.[60–62] Role-plays and case studies are useful strategies for preparing nurses to do assessments for abuse experiences. It is important that the time and place for the assessment is right, that the patient is medically stable, and that there is privacy. One example of creating privacy is taking a patient into a private cubicle to obtain a weight. Part of the training should focus on how to respond to the abuse. If the response is negative, it may cause the individual more harm. In response to disclosure, the nurse should be well prepared to respond in a supportive manner, indicating acceptance or belief, and providing validation, information, or other tangible aid. Waite and colleagues[62] provide a list of instruments that are commonly used for screening for trauma. They also provide an example of a focused inquiry about childhood abuse. They recommend beginning with the statement: "Please tell me about your childhood" and then following with precise questions about abuse/neglect. Next: "How was it living with your parents or the person(s) who raised you?" Then: "What is your favorite childhood memory?" followed by "What is your most awful memory from childhood?" and then "How were you punished in your home during your childhood?" They emphasize the importance of asking specific questions such as: "When you were a child, did an adult ever hurt or punish you in a way that left bruises, cuts, or scratches? Did anyone ever do something sexual that made you feel uncomfortable?"[62(pp56,57)]

The 2006 WHO report,[42] *Preventing Child Maltreatment: A Guide to Taking Action and Generating Evidence*, lists individual (parents and caregivers), child, relationship (family, friends, intimate partners, peers, community), and societal risk factors for child maltreatment and protective factors against child maltreatment.[42(pp14–16)] The factors are useful for assessing for potential abuse and to intervene before abuse occurs. For example, difficulty bonding is a risk factor that maternal child nurses may assess for during the labor and delivery and postpartum period.

How can Abuse be Stopped?

This quote from the 2006 WHO[42(p9)] report makes clear the need for social change to prevent violence:

Child maltreatment often occurs alongside other types of violence. For instance, child maltreatment by adults within the family is frequently found in the same settings as intimate partner violence. Maltreated children are themselves at increased risk in later life of either perpetrating or becoming the victims of multiple types of violence – including suicide, sexual violence, youth violence, intimate partner violence and child maltreatment. The same set of factors – such as harmful levels of alcohol use, family isolation and social exclusion, high unemployment, and economic inequalities – have been shown to underlie different types of violence. Strategies that prevent one type of violence and that address shared underlying factors therefore have the potential to prevent a number of different types of violence.

In countries with well-established universal health care, childcare, and greater economic equality, such as Japan (15%), the rates of lifetime physical and sexual partner violence against women were lower compared with countries with less support and greater economic inequality, such as Ethiopia (71%).[15] This distinction is not as clear in the finding that there is a low rate of assault during pregnancy (2%) in Australia, Cambodia, Denmark, and the Philippines.[17] Although Australia and Denmark have well-established universal health care, childcare, and greater economic equality, Cambodia and the Philippines do not, but their rates of assault during pregnancy are among the lowest. There is a need for further research to determine which factors in these countries are protective of pregnant women.

The work of Cohen and colleagues[48] shows that, even in the midst of trauma, effective help may prevent some further victimization. As noted earlier, in addition to improving children's IPV-related PTSD and anxiety, the 8-session, community-provided, trauma-focused CBT that they evaluated was associated with significantly fewer serious adverse events (reportable child abuse, child self-injury, and other serious problems requiring psychiatric hospitalization), compared with usual treatment. In the CBT sessions, they provided psychoeducation about trauma, developing individualized relaxation skills to manage stress, expressing and modulating feelings, and developing cognitive coping skills. They worked with the child to develop a narrative of the child's IPV experiences and helped correct maladaptive cognitions that became apparent through the narrative process. They worked on mastering responses to trauma reminders. During parent-child sessions, the child was encouraged to share the IPV experiences with the mother and there was work on discriminating between real danger and generalized fears. Although the focus of the research was on reducing mental health symptoms, this was associated with some prevention of further IPV.

Nurses working in emergency departments may have an opportunity to prevent violence in pregnant women. Kothari and colleagues[63] reviewed 3 years of prosecutor administrative reports, police incidence reports, and hospital medical records for a US countrywide sample of women (n = 964) who were assaulted by an intimate partner in 2000. In a comparison of perinatal and nonperinatal victims, they found that, after controlling for demographic and other factors, pregnant women were more likely to seek emergency department help in the 6 months before the assault (P<.01). It may be that assaults would be prevented by a concerted effort to provide all pregnant women who seek help in an emergency department with information about the cycle of violence and with information about establishing a safety plan.

How can nurses help?
It seems self-evident that the first treatment action would be to help the individuals victimized by IPV to leave the situation. Although the goal is establishing the safety of the individual being abused, the leaving and the time after leaving may present their own problems. Ford-Gilboe and colleagues[64] reviewed the literature about women's health issues as they leave abusive relations, and note that both improvements and deterioration in specific health function have been found in longitudinal studies of the physical and mental health consequences of IPV. Although women may experience relief and enhanced self-control, they may also experience multiple losses and life changes, as well as ongoing risk for violence from their former abusive partners. In addition, there are the challenges of facing ongoing health problems, economic hardships, changes in environment (including social relationships), and of getting help. To better understand the mediating influences that women's personal, social, and economic resources have on the relationship between the severity of past abuse experiences and current mental and physical health, they used data from a community sample of 309 Canadian women, who had experienced partner IPV within the last 3 years and had left their abusive partners, to evaluate 5 latent variables (IPV severity, personal resources, social resources, economic resources, and mental and physical health). They found that IPV severity was inversely correlated with personal, social, and economic resources, and that, when combined (but not independently), personal, social, and economic resources were significantly correlated with both mental and physical health, but that the direct effect of IPV on physical health was about 4 times as great as the direct effect of IPV on mental health. This research highlights the barriers women may face to leaving an abusive relationship and also the need for economic, social, and health care (mental and physical) resources for those who leave. The investigators note that the 2005 WHO[51] report identifies economic resources as the main factor in eradicating violence and emphasize that women with children and women with health problems may have particular difficulty finding and obtaining good jobs. They state that "interventions that reinforce women's strengths and support their control over decisions may be the key to developing a research agenda designed to promote the health and quality of life of women who have left abusive partners." Such interventions may be the key to providing effective clinical intervention for abused children, men, and women.

Providing those who are abused or at risk for abuse with information for contacting sources of support such as women's centers, crisis line phone numbers, and the United Way helpline (dial 2-1-1) are easy things that nurses in the United States can do. The US Department of Justice Office on Violence Against Women lists several national hotlines including the Domestic Violence Hotline (1-800-799-SAFE, 7233, or 1-800-787-3224, TTY). Despite their names, many women's centers provide help to men as well as to women and children. No matter where in the world nurses work, perhaps the most important things they can do are assess, listen with acceptance, discuss safety plans, and provide information about possible sources of help. For children and elders, there is a responsibility to report suspected abuse.

COSTS OF ABUSE

In 2003, investigators of a Centers for Disease Control and Prevention (CDC) report[65] estimated that the cost of IPV in the United States exceeded $5.8 billion each year. Most of this cost was for women's health care ($4.1 billion) and the remainder ($0.9

billion respectively) was for lost productivity and loss of lifetime earnings by victims of homicide. The investigators did not consider the effects of IPV on children in calculating the annual costs of IPV. The investigators of the WHO report,[3] *The Economic Dimensions of Interpersonal Violence*, note that, although there is overwhelming evidence for the high costs of interpersonal violence, there are few published studies evaluating economic evidence for interventions to prevent IPV, and, of those, most are from the United States. They suggest that part of the reason for the lack of such studies is that the prevalence of IPV is not well established, in part because reporting may violate social taboos.[3(p28)] Even with these constraints, the studies they reviewed uniformly showed that the cost of intervention was less than the amount saved by preventing abuse.

SUMMARY

Abuse affects everyone directly or indirectly. For those most seriously abused, physically, sexually, or psychologically, the results may be repeated abuse, chronic pain, and physical and emotional illnesses. For some, the result is death. Others go on to thrive. Although both males and females are abused at similar rates, males are more likely to experience physical assault and females are more likely to experience sexual assault. Males and females experience psychological abuse at the same rates and there is evidence that the effects of psychological abuse are at least as detrimental to long-term functioning as the effects of physical abuse.

An emerging finding that needs further research but has major implications for nursing interventions is that supportive parenting protects against the most serious mental health outcomes of abuse. Nurses may often be in positions to provide education to parents. Another finding that needs additional research, and also has implications for nursing interventions, is that those who identify what happened to them as abuse have fewer mental health symptoms. Assessing for abuse (personal safety), responding with acceptance to those who are abused, providing information about safety plans and sources of support, and reporting as necessary are important nursing interventions that should be supported with regular training sessions, including role-plays.

ACKNOWLEDGMENTS

The author is grateful to Dr Judith McFarlane for her ongoing support and mentoring.

REFERENCES

1. Merriam-Webster online dictionary. Available at: http://www.merriam-webster.com/dictionary/abuse. Accessed March 9, 2011.
2. World Health Organization. The World Health Report 2002 – reducing risks, promoting health life. 2002. Available at: http://www.who.int/whr/2002/en/. Accessed March 9, 2011
3. World Health Organization. The economic dimensions of interpersonal violence 2004. Available at: http://www.who.int/violence_injury_prevention/publications/violence/economic_dimensions/en/. Accessed March 14, 2011.
4. Kalisch BJ. Nursing actions in behalf of the battered child. Nurs Forum 1973;12(4):365–77.
5. Ortman E. Attachment behaviors in abused children. Pediatr Nurs 1979;5(4):25–9.

6. Riggs RS, Evans DW. Child abuse prevention–implementation within the curriculum. J Sch Health 1979;49(5):255–9.
7. Lieberknecht K. Helping the battered wife. Am J Nurs 1978;78(4):654–6.
8. Sammons LN. Battered and pregnant. MCN Am J Matern Child Nurs 1981;6(4): 246–50.
9. Phillips LR. Abuse and neglect of the frail elderly at home: an exploration of theoretical relationships. J Adv Nurs 1983;8(5):379–92.
10. Burgess AW, Holmstrom LL. The rape victim in the emergency ward. Am J Nurs 1973;73(10):1740–5.
11. Holmstrom LL, Burgess AW. Assessing trauma in the rape victim. Am J Nurs 1975;75(8):1288–91.
12. McFarlane J, Parker B, Soeken K. Abuse during pregnancy: associations with maternal health and infant birth weight. Nurs Res 1996;45(1):37–42.
13. Shay-Zapien G, Bullock L. Impact of intimate partner violence on maternal child health. MCN 2010;35(4):206–12.
14. Oyunbileg S, Samburzul N, Udval N, et al. Prevalence and risk factors of domestic violence among Mongolian women. J Womens Health 2009;18(11): 1873–80.
15. Garcia-Moreno C, Jansen HA, Ellsberg M, et al. Prevalence of intimate partner violence: findings from the WHO multi-country study on women's health and domestic violence. Lancet 2006;368:1260–9.
16. Breiding MJ, Black MC, Ryan GW. Prevalence and risk factors of intimate partner violence in eighteen U.S. states/territories, 2005. Am J Prev Med 2008;34(2): 112–8.
17. Devries KM, Kishor S, Johnson H, et al. Intimate partner violence during pregnancy: analysis of data from 19 countries. Reprod Health matters 2010;18(36): 158–70.
18. McFarlane J. Abuse during pregnancy: the horror and the hope. AWHONNS Clin Issues Pernat Womens Health Nurs 1993;4(3):350–62.
19. Abramsky T, Watts CH, Garcia-Moreno C, et al. What factors are associated with recent intimate partner violence? Findings from the WHO multi-country study on women's health and domestic violence. BMC Public Health 2011;11:109.
20. Li Q, Kirby RS, Sigler RT, et al. A multilevel analysis of individual, household, and neighborhood correlates of intimate partner violence among low-income pregnant in Jefferson County, Alabama. Am J Public Health 2010;100(3):531–9.
21. Daigneault I, Hébert M, McDuff P. Men's and women's childhood sexual abuse and victimization in adult partner relationships: a study in risk factors. Child Abuse Negl 2009;33:638–47.
22. Ali TS, Asad N, Mogren I, et al. Intimate partner violence in urban Pakistan: prevalence, frequency, and risk factors. Int J Womens Health 2011;3:105–15.
23. O'Campo P, Caughy MO, Nettles SM. Partner abuse or violence, parenting and neighborhood influences on children's behavioral problems. Soc Sci Med 2010; 70:1404–15.
24. Rennison C, Planty M. Nonlethal intimate partner violence: examining race, gender, and income patterns. Violence Vict 2003;18(4):433–43.
25. Ciccetti D. Resilience under conditions of extreme stress: a multilevel perspective. World Psychiatry 2010;9:145–54.
26. Young AM, Grey M, Boyd CJ. Adolescents' experiences of sexual assault by peers: prevalence and nature of victimization occurring within and outside of school. J Youth Adolesc 2009;38:1072–83.

27. Silverman JG, McCauley HL, Decker MR, et al. Coercive forms of sexual risk and associated violence perpetrated by male partners of female adolescents. Perspect Sex Reprod Health 2011;43(1):60–5.
28. Begle AM, Hanson RF, Danielson CK, et al. Longitudinal pathways of victimization, substance use, and delinquency: findings from the national survey of adolescents. Addict Behav 2011;36(7):682–9.
29. Senn RE, Carey MP. Child maltreatment and women's adult sexual risk behavior: childhood sexual abuse as a unique risk factor. Child Maltreat 2010;15(4): 324–35.
30. Messman-Moore T, Walsh KL, DiLillo D. Emotion dysregulation and risky sexual behavior in revictimization. Child Abuse Negl 2010;34:967–76.
31. Walsh K, Blaustein M, Knight WG, et al. Resiliency factors in the relation between childhood sexual abuse and adulthood sexual assault in college-age women. J Child Sex Abus 2007;16(1):1–17.
32. McKinney CM, Caetano R, Ramisetty-Miller S, et al. Childhood family violence and perpetration and victimization of intimate partner violence: findings from national population-based study of couples. Ann Epidemiol 2009; 19(1):25–32.
33. Farris C, Treat TA, Viken RJ, et al. Sexual coercion and the misrepresentation of sexual intent. Clin Psychol Rev 2008;28:48–66.
34. Vogt D, Bruce TA, Street AE, et al. Attitudes toward women and tolerance for sexual harassment among reservists. Violence Against Women 2007;13(9): 879–900.
35. Masho SW, Anderson L. Sexual assault in men: a population-based study of Virginia. Violence Vict 2009;24(1):98–110.
36. Romito P, Pomicino L, Lucchetta C, et al. The relationships between physical violence, verbal abuse and women's psychological distress during the postpartum period. J Psychosom Obstet Gynaecol 2009;30(2):115–21.
37. Garabedian MJ, Lain KY, Hansen WF, et al. Violence against women and postpartum depression. J Womens Health 2011;20(3):447–53.
38. Ludermir AB, Lewis G, Valongueiro SA, et al. Violence against women by their intimate partner during pregnancy and postnatal depression: a prospective cohort study. Lancet 2010;376(9744):903–10.
39. Ackerson LK, Subramanian SV. Intimate partner violence and death among infants and children in India. Pediatrics 2009;124:e878–89.
40. Rico E, Fenn B, Abramsky T, et al. Associations between maternal experiences of intimate partner violence and child nutrition and mortality: findings from demographic and health surveys in Egypt, Honduras, Kenya, Malawi and Rwanda. J Epidemiol Community Health 2011;65:360–7.
41. Silverman JG, Decker MR, Gupta J, et al. Maternal experiences of intimate partner violence and child morbidity in Bangladesh. Arch Pediatr Adolesc Med 2009;163(8):700–5.
42. World Health Organization. Preventing child maltreatment: a guide to taking action and generating evidence (pdf 867 kb). 2006. Available at: http://www. who.int/mediacentre/news/releases/2006/pr57/en/index.html. Accessed March 7, 2011.
43. Finkelhor D, Ormrod R, Turner H, et al. School, police, and medical authority involvement with children who have experienced victimization. Arch Pediatr Adolesc Med 2011;165(1):9–15.
44. Maugh D, Moore SC. Dimensions of child neglect: an exploration of parental neglect and its relationship with delinquency. Child Welfare 2010;89(4):47–65.

45. Turner HA, Finkelhor D, Hamby SL, et al. Specifying type and location of peer victimization in a national sample of children and youth. J Youth Adolesc 2011; 40(8):1052–67.
46. Knutson JF, Lawrence E, Taber SM, et al. Assessing children's exposure to intimate partner violence. Clin Child Fam Psychol Rev 2009;12:157–73.
47. Dubowitz H, Kim J, Black MM, et al. Identifying children at high risk for a child maltreatment report. Child Abuse Negl 2011;35:96–104.
48. Cohen JA, Mannarino AP, Iyengar S. Community treatment of posttraumatic stress disorder for children exposed to intimate partner violence. Arch Pediatr Adolesc Med 2011;165(1):16–21.
49. Breiding MJ, Ziembroski JS. The relationship between intimate partner violence and children's asthma in 10 US states/territories. Pediatr Allergy Immunol 2011; 22:e95–100.
50. Van Harmelen AL, van Tol MJ, van der Wee NJA, et al. Reduced medial prefrontal cortex volume in adults reporting childhood emotional maltreatment. Biol Psychiatry 2010;68:832–8.
51. World Health Organization. Multi-country study on women's health and domestic violence against women. 2005. Available at: http://www.who.int/gender/violence/who_multicountry_study/en/. Accessed March 10, 2011.
52. Wilson HW, Widom CS. Pathways from childhood abuse and neglect to HIV-risk sexual behavior in middle adulthood. J Consult Clin Psychol 2011;79(2):236–46.
53. Bonomi AE, Anderson ML, Reid RJ, et al. Medical and psychosocial diagnoses in women with a history of intimate partner violence. Arch Intern Med 2009;169(18): 1692–7.
54. Wuest J, Merritt-Gray M, Ford-Gilboe M, et al. Chronic pain in women survivors of intimate partner violence. J Pain 2008;9(11):1049–57.
55. Taft CT, Resick PA, Watkins LE, et al. An investigation of posttraumatic stress disorder and depressive symptomatology among female victims of interpersonal violence. J Fam Violence 2009;24(6):407–15.
56. Woods SJ, Wineman NM, Page GG, et al. Predicting immune status in women from PTSD and childhood and adult violence. ANS Adv Nurs Sci 2005;28(4): 306–19.
57. Wuest J, Ford-Gilboe M, Merritt-Gray M, et al. Abuse-related injury and symptoms of posttraumatic stress disorder as mechanisms of chronic pain in survivors of intimate partner violence. Pain Med 2009;10(4):739–47.
58. Tucker PM, Pfefferbaum B, North CS, et al. Physiologic reactivity despite emotional resilience several years after direct exposure to terrorism. Am J Psychiatry 2007;164:230–5.
59. Clements CM, Ogle RL. Does acknowledgement as an assault victim impact postassault psychological symptoms and coping? J Interpers Violence 2009; 24(10):1595–614.
60. Gregory A, Ramsay J, Agnew-Davies R, et al. Primary care identification and referral to improve safety of women experiencing domestic violence (IRIS): protocol for a pragmatic cluster randomized controlled trial. BMC Public Health 2010;10(54). Available at: http://www.biomedcentral.com/1471-2458/10/54.
61. Manchester A. Asking about and assessing for family violence – part of nurse's caring role. Kai Tiaki. Nurs N Z 2007;13(10):10–1.
62. Waite R, Gerrity R, Arango R. Assessment for and response to adverse childhood experiences. J Psychosoc Nurs 2010;48(12):53–60.
63. Kothari CL, Cerulli C, Marcus S, et al. Perinatal status and help-seeking for intimate partner violence. J Womens Health 2009;18(10):1639–46.

64. Ford-Gilboe M, Wuest J, Varcoe C, et al. Modelling the effects of intimate partner violence and access to resources on women's health in the early years after leaving an abusive partner. Soc Sci Med 2009;68:1021–9.

65. Centers for Disease Control and Prevention (CDC). Costs of intimate partner violence against women in the United States. 2003. Available at: http://www.cdc.gov/violenceprevention/pub/IPV_cost.html. Accessed March 18, 2011.

Child Abuse

MaryAnn Troiano, DNP, RN, APRN*

KEYWORDS

- Child abuse • Shaken baby syndrome • Diagnostic imaging
- NICE guidance • Parent-child interaction therapy

EPIDEMIOLOGY

In 2008, the US state and local child protective services (CPS) received 3.3 million reports of children being abused or neglected. Of these children, 71% were classified as victims of child neglect, 16% as victims of physical abuse, 9% as victims of sexual abuse, and 7% as victims of emotional abuse.[1] A non-CPS study estimated that 1 in 5 US children experience some form of child maltreatment: approximately 1% victims of sexual assault, 4% victims of child neglect, and 12% victims of emotional abuse. Rates of victimization were higher in several races. In 2008, African American children averaged 16.6 per 1000 children, American Indian or Alaska Native averaged 13.9 per 1000 children, and multiracial averaged 13.8 per 1000 children. In 2008, an estimated 1740 children aged 0 to 17 years died of abuse and neglect at a rate of 2.3 per 100,000 children. Of these children died, 39% were non-Hispanic white, 30% African American, and 16% Hispanic.[1]

Infants and young children (0 to 3 years old) suffer higher rates of abuse than older children. The rate of abuse is 16.4 per 1000 children for infants and young children versus 12.4 per 1000 children for all ages. These statistics include nondomestic forms of child abuse, including abuse by nonparent caregivers, teachers, neighbors, and strangers.[1] Parents are the perpetrators in 80% of child abuse cases. Girls are 4 times as likely to be sexually abused as are boys. Every year, approximately 1500 American children die of physical abuse or neglect, and 79% of the involved children are younger than 4 years.[1]

The World Health Organization includes neglect and commercial exploitation of children in its definition of child abuse, which includes human rights verbiage about the dignity of the child, abuse of trust, and responsibility of the adult.[2] Neglect represents 60% of the child abuse cases.

Shaken baby syndrome is the leading cause of death in abusive head trauma cases, with an estimated 1200 to 1400 children injured or killed by shaking each year in the United States. The estimate is that more than 300 babies a year die of shaken baby

Monmouth University, Marjorie K. Unterberg School of Nursing and Health Studies, 400 Cedar Avenue, West Long Branch, NJ 07764-1898, USA
* 35 Melrose Terrace, Middletown, NJ 07748.
E-mail address: mtroiano@monmouth.edu

Nurs Clin N Am 46 (2011) 413–422
doi:10.1016/j.cnur.2011.08.009   **nursing.theclinics.com**
0029-6465/11/$ – see front matter © 2011 Elsevier Inc. All rights reserved.

syndrome in the United States. Approximately 25% of all shaken baby syndrome/abuse head trauma victims die of their injuries, whereas 80% of those who survive suffer permanent disability, such as severe brain injury, cerebral palsy, mental retardation, behavioral disorders, and impaired motor and cognitive skills. The long-term medical costs of the survivors of shaken baby syndrome average $300,000 to $1,000,000.[3] Babies, especially newborns to 4-month olds, are at the greatest risk for injury from shaken baby syndrome. Inconsolable crying is the major trigger for shaken baby syndrome. Most perpetrators are by incidence father of the victim followed by child care providers, boyfriend of the mother, and mother of the victim.[3]

Child sexual abuse is an international phenomenon. It occurs in every culture and race, every religious sect, every socioeconomic tier, and at every educational level. An estimated 150,000 cases of child sexual abuse are substantiated by CPS agencies in the United States each year, for a rate of 1.1 cases per 1000 children. Approximately 30% of girls and 15% of boys experience some type of sexual abuse in childhood. Approximately 1 in 4 girls and 1 in 6 boys are sexually abused before their 18th birthday.[4]

Child sexual abuse is always for the benefit of the abuser, generally without regard for the reactions or choices of the child and the effects of the behavior on the child. In the United States, the annual number of reported cases of child sexual abuse is about 90,000, and 90% of cases go unreported because children are afraid to tell anyone what happened to them and the legal procedure for validating child sexual abuse is complex. Worldwide child abuse is experienced by approximately 20% of female and 10% of male children. About 60% of perpetrators of child sexual abuse are nonrelative acquaintances of the child. A friend of the family, neighbor, child care person, teacher, or coach can be the perpetrator. About 30% of perpetrators of child sexual abuse are relatives of the child, such as a parent, stepparent, grandparent, sibling, cousin, or other relative. Stranger perpetrators account for approximately 10% of child sexual abuse cases. Women are perpetrators in about 12% of the cases reported against boys and about 6% of the cases reported against girls. Men are the usual perpetrators against both girls and boys. Homosexual men are not more likely to sexually abuse children than other men are.[5]

FACTORS AFFECTING CHILD ABUSE

Children at risk for child maltreatment are those (a) who are from a family in which violence of the intimate partner is present (these children are at greater risk for physical and psychological abuse and child neglect[6]; (b) who are younger than 4 years (these children are at the greatest risk for severe injury and death); (c) who live in communities with a high level of violence and one that accepts child abuse; and (d) who live in families with great stress, such as from substance abuse, poverty, and chronic illness, and who do not have nearby friends or relatives who can provide support and assistance.[7]

There are 4 types of attitudes and behaviors seen in abusive or neglecting parents. First, there is an inappropriate parental expectation of the child. The second is a failure of empathy between parent and child or an inability of the parent to understand and participate in the child's emotional experience and ideas. The third is a placement of inherent value on the use of physical punishment. Fourth, abusive or neglecting parents may reverse the parent-child roles and see children as the source of family comfort and happiness.[8] All these attitudes and behaviors are predictors of child abuse.

Child abuse risks include male perpetrator, low self-esteem of perpetrator, and low levels of empathy and impulse control among perpetrators. Low educational attainment of the perpetrator is a risk factor of child sexual abuse but not of physical abuse. Intimate personal violence seems to increase the risk of physical violence toward children. Children with mental or physical disabilities are at greater risk for physical abuse. Communities that have an increased ethnic social network have lower child abuse rates, even in impoverished neighborhoods.[2]

In babies with shaken baby syndrome, those younger than 1 year and until 5 years of age are at risk and 2- to 4-month olds who are small in relation to the adult who picks them and shakes them are at the highest risk. At this age, a baby cries more frequently and longer than older babies. Inconsolable crying is one of the main reasons cited for shaking a baby. Factors that place a baby at risk include infants born prematurely, having a disability, and of a multiple birth and more often male. The parents or caregivers who abused these infants become frustrated with the infants crying, are usually tired, have limited anger management or coping skills, have decreased social support, are young-aged parents, and have an unstable family environment.[9]

DEFINITIONS
Child Physical Neglect

Physical neglect is depriving a child of the basic necessities of life. It is frequently defined as the failure of a parent or other person with the responsibility of providing the child with adequate food, proper clothing, shelter, hygiene, and medical or dental care.[10] Approximately 24 states, including the District of Columbia, American Samoa, Puerto Rico, and the Virgin Islands, include failure to educate the child as required by law in their definition of neglect. Seven states specifically define medical neglect as failing to provide any special medical treatment or mental health care needed by the child. In addition, 4 states define medical neglect as the withholding of medical treatment or nutrition from disabled infants with life-threatening conditions.[11] Dental neglect, as defined by the American Academy of Pediatric Dentistry, is the "willful failure of parent or guardian to seek and follow through with treatment necessary to ensure a level of oral health essential for adequate function and freedom from pain and infection." Dental neglect includes dental caries especially nursing caries, chipped or broken teeth, periodontal disease, and malformation of the teeth.[12]

Munchausen syndrome by proxy refers to a parent who repeatedly brings a child to a health care facility and reports symptoms of illness when, in fact, the child is well. Two classic findings of the syndrome are always present: first, the symptoms are not easily detected by physical examination, only by history; second, the symptoms are present only when the abuser is providing care and disappears when care is provided by another person.[13] The child's clinical symptoms may depend on the medical knowledge or sophistication of the parents. The parents may force a child to ingest medications or substances that induce vomiting and diarrhea, lethargy, and sleepiness. The skin may be burned, dyed, tattooed, lacerated, or punctured to stimulate acute or chronic skin lesions. Provision of intravenous lines during hospitalization may provide an opportunity for injection of infectious agents from feces, toxins, and pharmacologic agents.[14] This syndrome can occur for years and is associated with the death of infants and young children.

Child Emotional Neglect

Emotional neglect is the omission of basic nurturing, acceptance, and caring essential for healthy personal development. The caregiver ignores or treats the child as a nonentity. Emotional neglect is difficult to assess and can be subtle. The child usually suffers with self-esteem issues. Emotional neglect covers all socioeconomic families.[10]

Child Emotional Abuse

Emotional abuse involves extreme debasement of feelings and may result in the child feeling inadequate, inept, uncared for, and worthless. Victims of emotional abuse learn to hide their feelings to avoid incurring additional scorn.[10] The child may feel rejected and unwanted and suffers from lack of affection and physical touch. All states except Georgia, Washington, the District of Columbia, American Samoa, Guam, the Northern Mariana Islands, Puerto Rico, and the Virgin Islands include emotional maltreatment as part of their definitions of abuse or neglect. Approximately 32 states, including the District of Columbia, the Northern Mariana Islands, and Puerto Rico, provide specific definitions of emotional abuse or mental injury to a child. Typical language used in these definitions is "injury to the psychological capacity or emotional stability of the child as evidenced by an observable or substantial change in behavior, emotional response, or cognition" or as evidenced by "anxiety, depression, withdrawal, or aggressive behavior."[15]

Physical Abuse

Bruising is the most common physical sign of abuse. In young active children, normal bruising occurs. The obvious signs of accidental bruising occur on the knees and the anterior tibial area. Children routinely fall; so the bruised areas are the forehead, lower arms and elbows, hips, and spine. Red flags would be bruises over the upper arms, thighs, trunk, genitalia, and buttocks. Areas that are easily exposed include a child's hand, cheek, ears, and neck. The age of the child is another indicator of physical abuse. A perambulatory child with a single soft tissue injury should be investigated. Toddlers are known for running and not looking; so it is not unusual to have accidental bruising on their head and face but would be an indication of abuse in babies and school-aged children. The shape of the bruise is important, for it can give an indication of the object used in the physical abuse. The most commonly used instrument for physical abuse is the hand. Other instruments, such as belts, paddles, shoes, household gadgets, and electrical cords, will leave specific marks.[16]

Any bite mark should raise a suspicion of child abuse. Bite marks should be suspected when ecchymoses, abrasions, or lacerations are found in elliptical or ovoid patterns. Human bites compress flesh and can cause abrasions, contusions, and lacerations but rarely avulsions of tissue. An intercanine distance of more than 3.0 cm is suspicious of an adult human bite. They may be visualized more clearly 2 to 3 days after the injury because of decreased edema and surrounding erythema.[17]

Thermal injuries constitute about 10% of injuries to physically abused children and 5% of those who are sexually abused. The burns range from scalds to pattern burns. Fourteen percent of all pediatric scalds are related to abuse, whereas 28% to 45% of scalds are because of tap water. Immersion burns tend to be symmetric and have clear lines of demarcation, referred to as tide marks.[18] The immersion burns usually have uniform burn depth and involve the buttocks, perineum, and lower extremities. Several marks can be made by forced immersion.[19] Stocking and glove burns occur when a child's hands and/or feet are forcibly immersed in hot water, resulting in symmetric, circumferential, and well-demarcated burns. Zebra stripes are because of sparing of the flexural creases secondary to the body's flexed position in the hot liquid.[19] Donut-hole sparing occurs when the child's buttocks are pressed against a bathtub, which is relatively cooler than the water in it. These are highly suspicious of physical abuse.[19] When a child accidentally falls into a tub, the child has burn marks on the palms of the hands and splash marks on the face and chest. If a child is immersed in a hot tub, the dorsal aspect of the hands are involved.

Contact burns may be made by flames or a hot solid objective. Flame burns are characterized by extreme depth and are relatively well defined compared with accidental flame burns. Cigarette and iron burns are the most frequent types of contact burns. Cigarette burns are common and frequently leave blister formations on the back and buttocks. There can be multiple burns in a circular pattern on the skin. Accidental burns are usually shallower, irregular, and less well defined than deliberate burns. The abuser can use items that cause branding. Branding injuries usually mirror the objects that cause the burn, such as curling irons, pans, or steam irons.[20]

Shaken baby syndrome is the vigorous shaking of an infant or a child up to 5 years of age. With as few as 5 seconds, the baby can sustain neck, spine, eye, and brain injuries. Infants' heads are relatively large compared with their bodies and their neck. Shaking can slam the brain against the skull repeatedly, causing brain contusions (bruising), swelling, pressure, and bleeding. Tearing of meningeal vessels that run along the brain's exterior can cause bleeding, leading to permanent brain damage or death.[21] The child can develop whiplash injuries to the muscles of the neck. Hematomas, rib fractures, and retinal detachment are commonly seen in shaken babies.[21] Although there may not be outward bruising, the patient may present with behavioral symptoms. These symptoms may include lethargy, irritability, decreased appetite, vomiting, and, in severe cases, unconsciousness or coma.[21] The patient may present with seizure activity.

Sexual Abuse

Sexual abuse is the sexual activity between an adult and a child who cannot legally give consent. The Federal Child Abuse Prevention and Treatment Act defines sexual abuse as "the employment, use, persuasion, inducement, enticement, or coercion of any child to engage in, or assist any other person to engage in, any sexually explicit conduct or simulation of such conduct for the purpose of producing a visual depiction of such conduct; or the rape, and in cases of caretaker or inter-familial relationships, statutory rape, molestation, prostitution, or other form of sexual exploitation of children, or incest with children."[22]

The most important aspect of sexual abuse is not only the physical signs but also the history that the child states. If allowed to speak or draw, a child's report is usually truthful. Children may present with multiple nonspecific problems, such as a return to bedwetting, abdominal discomfort or pain, sleep disturbances, and nightmares. Physically, the most important aspect is to know the anatomy of the male and female child. The female child may present with bleeding, swelling, pain, or itching of the vagina, anus, mouth, and/or throat. The child may also present with odorous vaginal discharge; cuts and bruises; torn, stained, or bloody clothing; or difficulty in walking or sitting. The child who has gone through menarche should be observed for pregnancy.[5,8,23] The male child may present with semen in the mouth, in the rectum/anal canal, or on his clothes. An injured penis, rectum, anal canal, or scrotum with cuts and bruises, and torn, stained, or bloody clothes may be other presenting factors. The male child may also present with bleeding or bruising around the mouth or throat and increased signs of physical abuse.[23] Sexually transmitted infections highly indicate both male and female sexual abuse.

SCREENING

The most important screening tool is the history. A careful history detailing the events leading to the child's presentation to the emergency room or health care provider's office should be elicited.[8] The child should be interviewed alone and away from the parents or the suspected perpetrators.[8] The interviewer should use open-ended questions that are age appropriate and developmentally appropriate.[8,24] The interviewer should provide paper for a child to draw on to illustrate what happened to her/him.[8,24] The illustration may represent a suspected offender and the child perception of what has occurred and any injuries sustained.[24] A multidisciplinary team should be involved, and a witness to any interaction between the interviewer and the child should be present to prevent any bias.

A complete physical examination with normal growth and developmental status should be performed.[8] The practitioner needs to observe the child's affect, verbal and nonverbal responses, and the interaction with the parents. In sexual abuse cases, a careful examination of the genitals and anus should be performed.[8]

In child physical abuse cases, diagnostic testing should include tests that identify bruising and bleeding. These tests would include a complete blood count, a platelet count, a prothrombin time, a partial thromboplastin time, an international normalized ratio, and a bleeding time. These tests may also indicate an underlying bleeding disorder.[8]

Diagnostic imaging plays an important role in screening infants and young children. Infants and young children cannot describe their abuse, and symptoms such as vomiting, fever, lethargy, seizures, or coma are nonspecific to assault and alone do not constitute strong indications for child abuse screening.[25] In the presence of head injuries or bruising of the face, neck, or chest—particularly when inconsistent with the infant or child's presenting injury or the history of the injury as provided by the parent—these may indicate child abuse.[25] Unexplained injuries, particularly head injuries, bone fractures, bruising of the neck or face, burns, and delayed care seeking by parents, are all suggestive of child abuse.[25] For traumatic brain injuries and head, neck, and facial assault injuries, the skeletal survey imaging for fracture histories than a questionnaire is used.[25] The American College of Radiology (ACR) has issued guidelines on skeletal surveys for child battering and other indications. According to the ACR guidelines, detailed skeletal surveys with centered views at the joints and brain imaging with computed tomography or magnetic resonance imaging are indicated for any suspected child battering involving a patient younger than 2 years.[26] Some authors recommend a repeat skeletal survey 10 to 15 days after initial imaging to allow assessment of fracture healing.[26] No change in fractures suggests nontraumatic origins. Skeletal surveys are not generally used for children aged 5 years and older.[25]

Diagnostic tests in sexual abuse cases should consist of oral, urethral, vaginal, and rectal cultures. An oral, rectal, and vaginal examination should be performed for the detection of sexually transmitted diseases and swabs for prostatic acid phosphatase for the presence of semen.[8,13] Serum testing should be done for human immunodeficiency virus and syphilis, and for female children, a pregnancy test should be performed if she has undergone menarche.[8,13] Stool guaiac tests for occult blood may indicate rectal trauma. A rape kit should be performed on both genders to collect any forensic evidence (semen, pubic hair, and tissue samples for DNA.[13] A photocolposcopic examination may identify cervical/vaginal injuries.

PSYCHOSOCIAL ISSUES

Psychological/behavioral indicators of childhood abuse include a regression to behavior of a younger age, such as bedwetting, thumb sucking, whining, or clinging to parents.[13,23] They may appear uncharacteristically sad or withdrawn, or they may be angry and aggressive.[8,23] They may have problems in school, such as acting out or difficulty with schoolwork or concentrating.[23] They may have sleep problems, such as bad dreams, fear of the dark, or insomnia.[5,23] They may complain of recurring stomach aches or headaches when there is no reasonable explanation for the ailments.[13,23]

Sexually abused children often feel that they have done something wrong and are fearful that their family will reject them.[22] They may also fear the abuser and that their parent will do something to the abuser which will send the parent to jail and away from the child.[22] They often blame themselves and feel confused about the sexual abuse. Depression and isolation can last for some time. A child who is the victim of prolonged sexual abuse usually develops low self-esteem, a feeling of worthlessness, and an abnormal or a distorted view of sex.[5] The child may become withdrawn and mistrustful of adults and can become suicidal.[5] Some children who have been sexually abused have difficulty relating to others except on sexual terms. They may set fires, destroy personal possessions, exhibit sexual behavior inappropriate for their age, become self-destructive, or threaten suicide. Some sexually abused children become child abusers or prostitutes or have other serious problems when they reach adulthood.[23] Often the severe emotional damage to abused children does not surface until adolescence or even later, when many abused children become abusing parents. An adult who was abused as a child often has trouble establishing lasting and stable personal relationships. These men and women may have trouble with physical closeness, touching, intimacy, and trust as adults. They are also at higher risk for anxiety, depression, substance abuse, medical illness, and problems at school or work.[22]

EDUCATION

Health care providers should be aware of their state's mandate for reporting child abuse. All 50 states have a child protection ordinance mandating that professionals who come in contact with children report cases of suspected abuse to the local CPS agency.[27]

The National Institute for Health and Clinical Excellence (NICE) guidance on when to suspect child maltreatment covers the alerting features seen in children and young people in terms of physical, sexual, and emotional abuse, neglect, and fabricated or induced illness. It helps a practitioner to delineate what is considered abuse from suspected child abuse. The NICE guidance prompts the practitioner to listen, observe, seek an explanation from the parent, and record the information.[28]

Prompt recognition of sexual abuse coupled with reporting of concerns to the appropriate CPS agency can assure safety for the child. All well-child appointments should include a few developmentally appropriate screening questions for sexual abuse.[29] The pediatric nurse practitioner should provide education regarding private parts and that no one should touch, tickle, kiss, or hurt their private parts. One should explain to the child that it is only all right to be examining their genitals today because they are having a checkup and their parent is present.[29]

Shaken baby syndrome is a great concern for forensic nurses. Accurate diagnosis and treatment are essential. Forensic nurses should understand the history of shaken baby syndrome and the physical manifestations that may be caused by shaking.[30] Forensic nurses should educate medical staff on the physical manifestations that can ensue from shaken baby syndrome, educate parents on the effects shaking can have on their child, and continue research and investigation into the various injuries that are caused by shaking a baby.[30]

Several initiatives have occurred across the United States. In Fort Wayne, Indiana, a novel approach has been taken to fight forms of child abuse in the community. The Fort Wayne Children's Foundation, Inc, is a 509(a) (1) internal revenue service publicly supported organization that concentrates its energies to understanding and ridding our community of child abuse. It was formed to address a need for crisis care, programs, and education to combat child abuse and neglect in our community. The foundation has a legal action arm of a group of female attorneys, known as Kids Law. The union of the funding arm of the Fort Wayne Children's Foundation, Inc with the legal action of Kids Law has created a proactive program for child abuse abolition in Fort Wayne, Indiana.[27]

The Arkansas Center for Addictions Research, Education and Services provides comprehensive residential substance abuse prevention and treatment services to low-income pregnant women, mothers, and their children.[28] The center's main service is parenting classes. The mothers learn what behaviors are appropriate to expect of their children and how to practice positive discipline.[31]

The incredible years (IY) is considered to be one of the most effective interventions for reducing child conduct problems.[28] IY reduced children's physical aggression and parents' harsh parenting and increased parents' responsive parenting and their stimulation of their child's learning.[28]

Parent-child interaction therapy (PCIT) uses observation and direct audio feedback to the parent via headset to build parental competence in interacting with children whose behaviors are difficult and disruptive.[28] In the most compelling study of the effectiveness of PCIT in preventing physical abuse, Mark Chaffin and colleagues[32] showed that they could significantly improve parenting competence and lower the rates of repeated reports and reinvestigations for child abuse and neglect in Oklahoma.[28]

IMPLICATIONS

Child abuse can have a long-lasting and devastating effect on the growth and development of infants, children, and adolescents. Studies of abused and neglected children indicate that they have a higher rate of delayed intellectual development, poor school performance, aggressive behaviors, and social and relationship deficits compared with nonmaltreated children.[8] There is an increase in emotional difficulties, trusting relationships, suicide, and self-mutilation. There is clear evidence that children who have been maltreated have substantial problems with social interactions with peers. Children who were physically abused, in particular, have been noted to be physically aggressive and antisocial. Both abused and neglected children are at increased risk for juvenile delinquency, substance abuse, and self-destructive behaviors during adolescence.[8]

Every child is an individual, and not every child who is sexually abused will require ongoing mental health therapy. Infants and toddlers who are sexually abused would not be expected to have lasting memories of their sexual abuse and obviously are too young for mental health therapy. Preschool-aged, school-aged, and adolescent children who have been sexually abused should be referred to a mental health therapist with expertise in working with children who have been sexually abused for an assessment to determine the need for ongoing therapy.[29] Asymptomatic children can benefit from therapeutic intervention and education designed to prevent repeated sexual abuse, to normalize and clarify their feelings, and to educate regarding healthy sexual/personal boundaries.[29]

Early recognition and appropriate treatment is one of the most important factors in preventing further child abuse and maltreatment. Every practitioner should be educated on the signs and symptoms of child abuse. They should be aware of their mandated state laws and be prompt in identifying suspected child abuse or neglect. The referral to CPS is a necessity for the future well-being of the child.

REFERENCES

1. Centers for Disease Control and Prevention: Child maltreatment: facts at a glance sheet. 2010. Last updated April 14, 2010. Available at: http://www.cdc.gov/violencePrevention/Datasheet. Accessed March 31, 2011.
2. Tolan P, Gorman-Smith D, Henry D. Family violence. Annu Rev Psychol 2006;57: 577–83. In: Furlow B. Domestic violence. Radiol Technol 2010;82(2):133–53.
3. US National Library of Medicine. Shaken baby syndrome. Update date: March 14, 2009. Available at: www.nlm.nih.gov/medlineplus/ency/article/000004.htm. Accessed April 2, 2011.
4. Centers for Disease Control and Prevention: Understanding child maltreatment fact sheet. 2006. Updated April 14, 2011. Available at: http://www.cdc.gov/injury. Accessed April 14, 2011.
5. Golanty E, Edlin G. Sexual coercion and assault. In: Golanty E, Edlin G, editors. Human sexuality: the basics. Sudbury (MA): Jones and Bartlett Learning; 2012. p. 232–6.
6. English D, Marshall D, Stewart A. Effects of family violence on child behavior and health during early childhood. J Fam Violence 2003;18(1):43–57.
7. Centers for Disease Control and Prevention: Child maltreatment: risk and protective factors. 2008. Updated June 1, 2009. Available at: http://www.cdc.gov/injury. Accessed April 2, 2011.
8. Leventhal J. Abuse, neglect, violence. In: Rudolph C, Rudolph A, Lister G, et al, editors. Rudolph's pediatrics. 22nd edition. New York: McGraw Hill Medical; 2011. p. 137–53.
9. Preventing shaken baby syndrome: a guide for health departments and community-based organizations. Available at: http://www.cdc.gov/concussion/pdf./preventing-SBS-508-a-pdf. Updated July 15, 2008. Accessed April 6, 2011.
10. Landenburger K, Campbell J. Violence and human abuse. In: Stanhope M, Lancaster J, editors. Foundations of nursing in the community: community-oriented practice. 3rd edition. St Louis (MO): Mosby; 2010. p. 462–82.
11. Federal Child Abuse Prevention and Treatment Act (CAPTA). Available at: http://www.childwelfare.gov/systemwide/laws_policies/. Accessed April 2, 2011.
12. American Academy of Pediatric Dentistry. Definition of dental neglect. Pediatr Dent 2003;25(Suppl):11–49.
13. Pillitteri A. Nursing care of the family in crisis: abuse and violence in the family. In: Maternal and child health nursing: care of the childbearing and childrearing family. 3rd edition. Philadelphia: Lippincott Williams and Williams; 2007. p. 1742–63.
14. Schreier H, Libow J. Munchausen syndrome by proxy: diagnosis and prevalence. Am J Orthopsychiatry 1993;63:318–21. In: Ermertcan A, Ertan P. Skin manifestations of child abuse. Indian J Dermatol Venereol Leprol July/Aug 2010:317–26.
15. Definitions of child abuse and neglect: summary of state laws. Available at: www.childwelfare.gov. Accessed April 6, 2011.
16. Ermertcan A, Ertan P. Skin manifestations of child abuse. Indian J Dermatol Venereol Leprol 2010;76(4):317–26.
17. Nuzzolese E, Lepore M, Montagna F, et al. Child abuse and dental neglect: the dental team's role in identification and prevention. Int J Dent Hyg 2009;7(2): 96–101.
18. Yeoh C, Nixon J, Dickson W, et al. Patterns of scald injuries. Arch Dis Child 1994; 7(12):156–8. Ermertcan A, Ertan P. Skin manifestations of child abuse. Indian J Dermatol Venereol Leprol 2010;76(4):317–26.

19. Kos L, Shwayder T. Cutaneous manifestations of child abuse. Pediatr Dermatol 2006;23(4):311–20.
20. US Department of Justice. Burn injuries in child abuse. Available at: www.missingkids.com/en.US/documents/burn_injuries.pdf. Accessed April 6, 2011.
21. US National Library of Medicine. Shaken baby syndrome. Available at: www.nlm.nih.gov/medlineplus/ency/article/000004.htm. Accessed April 2, 2011.
22. Children's Bureau. What is child abuse and neglect? Child welfare information gateway US Department of Health and Human Services, 2008. Available at: http://www.childwelfare.gov/pubs/factsheets/whatiscan.cfm. Accessed April 6, 2011.
23. American Academy of Child and Adolescent Psychiatry (2011) facts for families: child sexual abuse. Updated March 2011. Available at: http://aacap.org/page.ww?name=Child+Sexual+Abuse&section=Facts+for+Families. Accessed April 6, 2011.
24. Piperno F, DiBiasi S, Levi G. Evaluation of family drawings of physically and sexually abused children. Eur Child Adolesc Psychiatry 2007;16(6):389–97.
25. Degraw M, Hicks R, Lindberg D. Incidence of fractures among children with burns with concern regarding abuse. Pediatrics 2010;125:E295–9.
26. American College of Radiology. ACR practice guideline for skeletal surveys in children. Available at: www.acr.org/SecondaryMian.menuCategories/quality_safety/guidelines/pediatric/skeletalsurveys.apx. Updated 2006. Accessed April 3, 2011.
27. Cox J, Webber B, Joachim G. A community program to fight child abuse: the Fort Wayne Children's Foundation and Kids' Law. J Manipulative Physiol Ther 2007;30(8):607–13.
28. Barth R. Preventing child abuse and neglect with parent training: evidence and opportunities. Future Child 2009;19:95–118.
29. Hornor G. Child sexual abuse: consequences and implications. J Pediatr Health Care 2010;24(6):358–64.
30. Marz M. The physical manifestations of shaken baby syndrome. J Forensic Nurs 2009;5(1):26–30.
31. Connors N, Grant A, Crone C, et al. Substance abuse treatment for mothers: treatment outcomes and the impact of length of stay. J Subst Abuse Treat 2006;31(4):447–56.
32. Chaffin M, Silovsky JF, Funderburk B, et al. Parent-child interaction therapy with physically abusive parents: efficacy for reducing future abuse reports. J Consult Clin Psychol 2004;72(3):500–10.

"I know it shouldn't but it still hurts" Bullying and Adults: Implications and Interventions for Practice

Laura Kelly, PhD, PMHNP

KEYWORDS

- Workplace violence • Bullying cyberbullying • Adults
- Interventions

"I know it shouldn't but it still hurts: Bullying and Adults"

Sharon, a 35-year-old, recently divorced, public school teacher describes her entry into the world of technology. "I joined a social network to find old friends and to keep up with current ones. Everyone is doing it. I thought this is how people socialize today." She then relates that she was "de-friended" by a group of women that she went to high school with. "I have no idea what I did, they just dumped me, I feel like I am sixteen again." She describes that she spent 2 nights reviewing everything that she wrote to see if she somehow offended someone.

John is a 28-year-old, single, gay, social worker. He is an avid, frequent user of a popular social network. "It keeps me connected. I always know what is going on." One day he was visiting a coworker's homepage and there was a picture posted, with John's face attached to another person's body. The body was nude and holding a large bottle of liquor. The caption underneath said, "The fag can't hold his liquor." "I cried. How many people saw that picture?" He shared that his friend removed it and said it was "just a joke." John verbalizes that he now feels anxious in social settings.

Kevin, a 35-year-old, married father of two children is a police officer. He describes his immediate supervisor as a bully. "I'm a constant target of his craziness. The other guys tell me, 'you're it, it's your turn." Apparently, other officers have been verbally abused by this bully in the past. Kevin describes being told to do one thing and,

---

The author has nothing to disclose.

Marjorie K. Unterberg School of Nursing and Health Studies, Monmouth University, 400 Cedar Avenue, West Long Branch, NJ 07764, USA

E-mail address: lkelly@monmouth.edu

when it is done, being reprimanded for doing it. "And this guy is good. You should see the show he puts on for the big boss—he makes it look like I screwed up!" Kevin reports calling out sick and numerous other somatic complaints. He shares, "Secretly, I hope he finds a new victim. I don't want anyone else to suffer like I have, but I am at the end of my rope."

These examples are client scenarios from the author's clinical practice. Bullying is a national health problem affecting millions of children and adolescents. The literature is replete with articles examining bullying and cyberbullying of youth. Literature on bullying of adults is generally confined to workplace violence and harassment. No literature describes cyberbullying and adults.

There is an expectation that, as children mature into adults, bullying behavior will decrease.[1] As children mature and learn empathy, they are better able to understand how their actions can make other people feel. Society often views bullying as a problem of youth. There are many programs in place to educate young people about the effects of bullying. There are few such programs for adults.[2]

This creates a veil of silence for the adult victims of bullying. The victims also believe that this is a problem of childhood. Furthermore, bullied adults have a difficult time telling their stories and trying to make sense out of what is happening to them and why they are feeling as they do. They often blame themselves for their situation. This blame is validated by others who believe that the bullied are just thin-skinned, that the real world is tougher than the playground, and that victims or bullying targets should just grow up.

This article discusses workplace and cyberbullying of adults, identifies implications for nursing practice, and suggests interventions to identify and assist the victims of bullying.

WORKPLACE BULLYING

Workplace bullying is a big problem. According to recent research, 25% to 30% of the United States workforce are bullied or verbally abused sometime during their work lives.[3,4] If this many workers are being bullied, clearly it is not just a problem for a few overly sensitive or disgruntled employees.

Adult bullying at work is defined as situations in which employees are exposed to repeated, persistent, negative acts that are intimidating, malicious, and stigmatizing.[2] Victims usually report that they are unable to stop the behavior once it becomes an established mode of interaction.[5] Bullied workers generally perceive the abuse as intentional efforts to control, harm, or drive them from the workplace.[6]

Why Do Some Adults Become Workplace Bullies?

Workplace bullies often feel the need to be in control of all aspects of the work environment.[5] Bullies may also have an exaggerated sense of self, low self-esteem, or a lack of ability to feel remorse or guilt about inflicting harm on others.[7,8] Bullies who are unable to feel empathy were probably always bullies. They are the adult version of the playground bully. Attempting to gain self-esteem by hurting others is pathological and is painful to the victims of such abuse. The adult bully is unable to break the psychological cycle that he or she learned as a child and carries on that destructive behavior in their home, work, or social environment.[9]

Workplace Bullying Behaviors

Bullying behaviors in the workplace includes public name-calling, spreading of malicious rumors, increasing work pressures, sexual harassment, and physical abuse. The workplace is a natural environment for interpersonal conflicts and workplace bullying occurs because there is often competition and conflict between employees. Luzio-Lockett (1995) characterized the workplace as a group-oriented environment that is typified by "differences of opinions, a competition for power and territoriality, jealousy, prejudice, envy, and problematic group dynamics."[10(p12)]

Consequences of Workplace Bullying

Research on workplace bullying has identified many negative consequences to the bullying victim. They include poor mental and physical health, increased use of sick days, an increase in worker's compensation claims, and decreased productivity.[9] Psychosomatic illness is also a consequence,[11] as is a decrease in satisfaction in personal and professional relationships.[12]

CYBERBULLYING

Cyberbullying involves sending or posting harmful or cruel messages or images and using the Internet (eg, instant messaging, e-mails, chat rooms, social network sites) or other digital devices, such as cell phones.[13]

Social networking sites were first created for adults.[14] The number of adults using this technology is enormous. Cyberspace, although offering many opportunities to keep connected instantly, 24 hours a day, also enables quick and anonymous messages to potentially large audiences.

Why Do Some Adults Become Cyberbullys?

There may be many triggers for cyberbullying, such as relationship fights or break ups. Other triggers may be motivated by hate or bias because the victim is different in terms of race, religion, disability, sexual orientation, or body shape or size. Sometimes the motivation is simply entertainment. The bully is bored and posts hurtful things about someone else using the guise of making a joke. Often, cyberbullying is an outlet for adults who do not know how to deal with feelings of social frustrations.[15]

Cyberbullying can also become a way for an angry friend or ex-partner to retaliate. However, the bully may not have realized that technological retaliation can have far-reaching consequences. Pictures, texts, and e-mails are very hard to retrieve once they are launched into cyberspace. Impulsive bullies may hit the send button before thinking about the consequences of the action.

The prevalence of cyberbullying is increasing because people are more likely to say things online that they would not say face-to-face. Disinhibition, or a lack of restraint, including disregard for normal social conventions, is much easier when the bully does not have to see the victim. The technology acts as a buffer from the normal social cues. The bully may believe, because they cannot see the victim, that the negative actions are somehow less hurtful.[15]

Cyberbullying among adults is also likely to increase because adults are not receiving the formal education that children and adolescents are receiving in school regarding bullying and the dangers of technology. After treating middle-aged adults for many years, the author recognizes that they may not understand the far-reaching implications of the use of technology as well as younger adults who have been brought up in this advanced world of communication.

Cyberbullying Behaviors

Cyberbullying behaviors can be direct or indirect. Flaming is an indirect form of cyber-bullying that involves an argument between two people that includes rude language, insults, and threats.[16]

Direct cyberbullying can include exclusion and humiliation. Online exclusion occurs when victims are rejected from (de-friended) or left out of communications. Humiliation occurs when pictures (actual or manipulated) or negative, embarrassing messages are posted about someone else. Humiliation can also occur if a private message sent to one sender is forwarded to others or otherwise made public (outing).[17]

Consequences of Cyberbullying

Although there is no research on the impact that cyberbullying may have on adults, there are a few studies that identify the negative impact of cyberbullying on children and adolescents.

Raskauskas and Stolz (2007) observed that teenage cybervictims reported depression, sadness, hopelessness, and anxiety.[18] Kowalski and colleagues[19] (2008) showed that cybervictims had high levels of social anxiety and low self-esteem.

Although the clinical literature is lacking, there have been many reports of extremely negative consequences for those who are cybervictims. The most recent was the case of Tyler Clementi, the Rutgers University freshman who killed himself after his room-mate and another student videotaped him having sex and posted it for others to see.[19]

Another disturbing story was the case of Lori Drew who was the mother of a teenage girl. Lori created a fake persona of a teenage boy and a fake social network page and baited an ex-friend of her daughter. The other girl, Megan Meier, came to believe that the fake boy really cared for her and, after several months of an online relationship, the "boy" told Megan the world would be a better place without her. Megan killed herself the next day. Lori Drew was convicted of only a misdemeanor offense in this case.[5]

These are two examples in which adults were victims and the perpetrators. There are many more examples of adults engaging in cyberbullying. One only needs to peruse social network pages and observe the disturbing pictures and messages posted by many adults.

IMPLICATIONS FOR NURSING

Nurses assess patients every day for indications of violence or abuse. Although many nurses feel discomfort asking questions about abuse and violence of domestic partners, elders, and children, these subjects have become standard parts of nursing assessments. In the United States, there are laws that require reporting of certain types of abuse.

What is currently missing in nursing assessments is direct questioning of adults about bullying behaviors. Although nurses may ask if there is a history of physical, sexual, or verbal abuse, these questions do not generally address intimidation behaviors and cyberabuse.

Nurses need to recognize that the patient may feel embarrassed or ashamed by bullying. The societal message for the target of bullying is that they are at fault or, as adults, they "just need to get over it." This belief by the victim can be painful and psychologically distressing, especially if they cannot "just forget about it." It is the author's experience that shame and doubt can be pervasive feelings for the victim.

The nurse will most likely have more contact with the victims of bullying than the bullies themselves because the latter often do not see their behavior as problematic. Education about workplace bullying has become more a part of workplace culture in the last 10 years, as the problem has received a lot more attention. Cyberbullying needs to be added to education programs in the workplace and across college campuses so that young adults understand the problems and negative consequences of this type of violence.

INTERVENTIONS

The interventions presented are specifically for the victim or target of bullying because they are more likely than the bully to be identified by the nurse. The interventions, useful for both cyberbullying and workplace bullying are presented metaphorically because the author believes it is easier to remember the interventions when they are placed in a familiar context.

How to Avoid Being Eaten by Bears: Interventions for the Adult Target of Bullying Behavior

Keep food and trash in airtight containers
In the workplace Be cautious about the types of information you share with others. Although office friendships are common and important, be aware of boundaries, once crossed, may be used in ways that can show your vulnerabilities. Keep work friendships at a healthy distance. Save your intimacies for the people who are most important to you. You never know when a coworker may someday become a subordinate or supervisor.

In cyberspace No one needs to know what you are doing every second of the day. There is no need to post a message when you have run to the bathroom or have gone to a boring meeting. Remember, once sent, thousands of people have access. Be cautious about how much personal information you share. Even if the information is not written, pictures tell much about a person. Do not give ammunition to potential cyberbullies.

Keep a clean camp; get rid of old odors that might be clinging from past meals
In the workplace Be mindful of the moment. One must understand the past to learn how to manage present workplace situations; however, living in it can cause you to be unable to let go of difficult or painful situations. Go to work each day living in the present moment with the belief that things will be satisfactory. Although they may not be, at least you are headed into the day with positive self-talk that may protect you from bullying and make it easier to ask for help.

In cyberspace The past is called the past for a reason. Is it necessary to try to reconnect with old friends from high school? If the friends were that important, they would be in the present instead of in the past. Connecting with people from the past can cause old resentments, unresolved as a teenager, to resurface, bringing back bad feelings that were left behind long ago. This can leave you open to the bullying common to teenagers.

When walking in the woods, make a lot of noise; sing, clang pots, and, periodically, holler
In the workplace There are workplace policies against bullying. Do not tolerate it. Stop it when it starts. Remember, the bully is the problem. Tell the bully to stop as soon as a problem is perceived. Using "I" statements can help you feel powerful by taking responsibility for your feelings about a situation. A potential bullying situation can be defused quickly if you act quickly. One problem is that you is not always aware that you are being bullied and, by the time you are aware, the situation has gone on for

a long time. The first time you feel bullied, constructive confrontation in the form of "I" statements allow the bully to hear how you feels. If this stops the behavior, the problem is solved. If it does not, you need to follow workplace policies to protect yourself.

In cyberspace Social network sites have rules of conduct. If the bully refuses to remove pictures or posts that are inappropriate, contact the social networking site.

Avoid coming between the bear and its food or cubs at all costs; it is extraordinarily defensive and may attack if it feels threatened
In the workplace and in cyberspace Bullying back is not the answer. Engaging in the same behaviors as the bully, such as attacking the bully's vulnerabilities or the things they deem important, makes you a bully. It will also escalate the bully's behavior because they will become defensive when attacked.

If you see a bear, join others so you look bigger
In the workplace Bullies prey on those they believe are vulnerable. Run in a pack. This does not mean you have to agree with all of your coworkers, but getting along with them is important. Be transparent. Do not keep secrets. Do not get over-involved in the personal politics of the work environment. Work on getting along with others. Create a work environment where you are generally liked and respected. Bullies avoid people that do not seem vulnerable. This does not mean that you will not be bullied, but it does give you a support system if you are.

In cyberspace With groups of friends, share only information that you are comfortable with anyone knowing. Recognize a difference between your close, intimate friends and your online friends. Join groups where you share similar interests about general things. Personal, intimate topics should be shared face-to-face, not in cyberspace.

Carry bear-deterrent spray; if a bear gets too close, spray it in the face and slowly back away
In the workplace Adopt the "fool me once, shame on you; fool me twice, shame on me" philosophy. You should not wait until you are suffering from the psychological or physical consequences of chronic bullying. If you cannot resolve the bullying problem on your own, get help. You need to identify the policies and procedures at work or, if necessary, take legal action.

In cyberspace You should report the behaviors to the social networking site if the bully refuses to stop engaging in the adverse behaviors. This may not always be possible if the behaviors are those of exclusion or via e-mail or texting. When that is the case, you might choose to remove yourself from the situation by leaving cyberspace. Legal action is sometimes possible, depending on the bullying behaviors.

SUMMARY

Whereas bullying problems among children and adolescents are well documented in the clinical literature, little examines this phenomenon among adults. Nurses must begin to assess adult patients for this type of violence. Direct questions about being bullied at work or in cyberspace should be added to assessments. Questioning will help the bullying victim recognize that what they are going through is not acceptable and not their fault. It will also help identify patients who may need interventions beyond the treatment of the traumatic effects of bullying.

Although interventions for the victims are helpful, education is necessary for adults to understand the phenomenon of workplace violence and cyberbullying. Nursing research focused especially on cyberbullying will help create a body of knowledge so that the concept will be better defined and understood.

REFERENCES

1. Keashley L, Neuman J. Bullying in the workplace: its impact and management. Employee Right Employ Pol J 2005;8:335–73.
2. Lutgen-Sandvik P. The communicative style of employee abuse: generation and re-generation of workplace mistreatment. Manage Commun Q 2003;16:471–501.
3. Einarsen S, Hoel H, Zapf D, et al. The concept of bullying at work: the European tradition. In: Einarsen S, Hoel H, Zapf D, et al, editors. Bullying and emotional abuse in the workplace: international perspectives in research and practice. London: Taylor & Francis; 2003. p. 3–30.
4. Rayner C, Keashly L. Bullying at work: a perspective from Britain and North America. In: Fox S, Spector P, editors. Counterproductive work behavior: investigations of actors and targets. Washington, DC: American Psychological Association; 2005. p. 271–96.
5. Murray J. Workplace bullying in nursing: a problem that can't be ignored. Medsurg Nurs 2009;18(5):273–6.
6. Felblinger D. Incivility and bullying in the workplace and nurses' shame responses. J Obstet Gynecol Neonatal Nurs 2008;37(2):234–42.
7. Haynie D, Nansel T, Eitel P, et al. Bullies, victims and bully/victims: distinct groups of at risk youths. J Early Adolesc 2001;21(1):29–49.
8. Djurkovic N, McCormack D, Casimir G. The physical and psychological effects of workplace bullying and their relationship to intention to leave. International Journal of Organizational Theory and Behavior 2004;7:469–97.
9. Farrell A, Geist-Martin P. Communicating health: perceptions of wellness at work. Manag Comm Q 2005;18:543–92.
10. Luzio-Lockett A. Enhancing relationships within organizations an examination of a proactive approach to "bullying at work". J Early Adolescence 1995;7(1):12–22.
11. Feinberg T, Robeey N. Cyberbullying: school leaders cannot ignore but must understand the legal and psychological ramifications. Educational Digest 2009;26–31.
12. Ellison N, Steinfield C, Lampe C. The benefits of Facebook friends: social capital and college students' use of online network sites. J Computer Mediated Communication 2007;12(4):36–49.
13. Draa V, Sydney T. Cyberbullying: challenges and actions. Journal of Family and Consumer Science 2009;101(4):40–6.
14. Diamanduros T, Downs E, Jenkins S. The role of school psychoogists in assessment, prevention and intervention of cyberbullying. Psychol Schools 2008;45(8): 693–704.
15. Willard N. (2005). An educator's guide to cyberbullying and cyber threats. Available at: http://csriu.org/cyberbulying/pdf. Accessed March 17, 2011.
16. Foderaro L. Tyler Clementi's parents say they don't seek harsh punishment. New York Times. Available at: http://nytimes.com. Accessed March 23, 2011.
17. Meredith J. Combating cyberbullying: emphasizing education over criminalization. Federal Communications Law Journal 2010;63(1):311–40.
18. Raskauskas J, Stoltz A. Involvement in traditional and electronic bullying among adolescents. Dev Psychol 2007;43:564–75.
19. Kowalski R, Limber S. Electronic bullying among middle school students. J Adolesc Health 2007;41(6):S22–30.

Blind, Deaf, and Dumb: Why Elder Abuse Goes Unidentified

Sharon W. Stark, PhD, RN, APN-C, CFN

KEYWORDS

• Elder abuse • Prevalence • Implications

Elder abuse includes acts of physical, psychological, verbal, and financial abuses as well as abandonment and neglect. Elder abuse has no boundaries. It is not limited to elders living independently in their own homes being provided assistance by significant others, adult children, other family members, or friends as their informal caregivers. According to the National Center on Elder Abuse (2005), "Elder abuse is any knowing, intended, or careless act that causes harm or serious risk of harm to an older person—physically, mentally, emotionally, or financially."[1(p5)]

Elder abuse has the potential to occur in any senior care facility that elders frequent, whether in rehabilitation centers, long-term care facilities, nursing homes, and/or senior day care centers where they are cared for by formal caregivers. Children, family members, friends, and formal caregivers are prospective perpetrators of elder abuse. Sadly, perpetrators of abuse are often a relative who lives with an elder and has cared for the elder for a long period of time.[2–4]

AGING STATISTICS

As "baby boomers" continue to age, the number of elders in society continues to increase. In fact, by 2020, estimates indicate that 18% of the United States population will comprise elders and by 2050 elders will account for 25% of the population (United States Population Projections, 2008). The fastest growing segment in the United States is that of elders 85 years and older. In fact by 2030, the number of Americans older than 85 years will more than double.[4]

The United States is not alone in experiencing a rapidly expanding elderly population. The World Health Organization projects that the global population of elderly

The author has nothing to disclose.
Monmouth University, Marjorie K. Unterberg School of Nursing and Health Studies, 400 Cedar Avenue, West Long Branch, NJ 07764, USA
E-mail address: swstark@monmouth.edu

will double from 542 million in 1995 to 1.2 billion by 2025. Unfortunately, the potential for elder abuse is likely to increase proportionately, and its impact on public health will escalate.[5]

ELDER ABUSE PERVASIVENESS

Very few population-based studies have been conducted, therefore the extent of reports of elder abuse is limited. Estimates show that for every case of elder abuse or neglect that is reported, 4 to 5 are not. In fact, 84% of cases are never reported to any adult protective service agency.[1,4,6]

Between 4% and 6% of the elderly living at home have experienced some form of abuse. The United Nations Elder Population Division (2002) reported that from 1% to 35% of elders older than 65 years have or will experience some form of abuse by a person they trust.[7–9] The National Elder Mistreatment Study revealed that of the 7000 community-living elderly surveyed, approximately 10% reported at least one form of mistreatment in the past year.[10]

RISK FACTORS

Elder abuse risk factors cannot be isolated to individual circumstances. Rather, risks are a combination of factors that increase the likelihood that abuse will occur. Increasing physical and cognitive decline of the elderly that increases caregivers' responsibilities are common reasons for abusive behaviors among caregivers. Walsh and colleagues[11] explored the interrelationship between oppression and elder abuse. A literature review revealed that even though the popular belief is that males are more likely to be abusers and elderly women are more likely to be victims of abuse, there are conflicting reports regarding the gender of perpetrators and victims of elder abuse. Some studies showed that women committed over half of the cases of abuse or neglect, whereas men were more likely to commit physical, emotional, and financial abuse.[11]

Inadequate support systems, poor coping mechanisms, depression, substance abuse, greater perceived burden, and increased financial strain are reasons given for increased likelihood of elder abuse. Shared living space, social isolation, and mental illness of the caregiver also are reasons for caregivers to be abusive. Increasing age, multiple morbidities, greater physical and/or financial needs, dementia, social isolation, current or past abusiveness, and aggressiveness of elders needing care raises the likelihood that an elder will be abused.[5,12–14] The National Elder Mistreatment Study reported that the risk of elder mistreatment is higher for individuals who are in poor health, unemployed or retired, have low levels of social support, low household income, and/or have experienced a prior traumatic event.[15]

CULTURE AND SOCIETY

Definitions of abuse are as varied as culture and ethnic communities. The portrayal of elders as frail and weak devalues them, and diminishes their status and influence in families and society.[7,16] Elderly, widowed women are at risk of being abandoned and having their property seized in cultures where they have inferior social status.[7] Moreover, a common societal belief that what goes on in one's own home is private allows greater opportunity for abuse to go unreported. Cultural norms and beliefs about violence, social isolation, and language barriers also hinder reporting abuse among minorities.[11] Language barriers can make it difficult to distinguish abuse and/or neglect. It is important not to ignore abuse by attributing abuse to cultural differences, but it is as important to be sensitive to cultural differences so as not to mistake cultural traditions for abuse or neglect.[16] As young adults continue to migrate out of their cultural communities, elderly parents are left alone, without access to the care previously provided by their children.[7]

ELDER ABUSE LAWS

Internationally, some countries have developed sophisticated legal systems for reporting and prosecuting elder abuse cases, whereas other countries have very limited resources to protect the elderly from abuse. Laws that protect the elderly in countries that have such laws vary from country to country as well.[7]

In the United States, there are federal laws concerning domestic violence and child abuse, yet there are none specific for elder abuse. Less than 2% of federal funds for abuse prevention go toward elder abuse efforts, whereas 91% is earmarked for child abuse and 7% for domestic abuse, even though the risk for death is 300% higher among abused elderly than those who are not abused.[4] The Elder Justice Act was signed into law in 2010. It provides federal funds for adult protective services to test methods to better identify, respond to, and prevent elder abuse. The 2012 federal budget proposes $16.5 million in funding to undertake this effort.[17] Every state has elder abuse prevention laws and some form of reporting system, but there are inconsistencies between states regarding abuse definitions, services provided, who is covered by elder abuse laws, and mandatory reporting requirements of witnessed or suspected abuse. Such inconsistencies make it difficult to regulate or standardize elder abuse services. Without standardized definitions of elder abuse and abuse-reporting systems, it will continue to be challenging to accurately assess its prevalence and determine how to stimulate solutions.[18,19]

HEALTH SERVICES

Health services and social programs aimed at the elderly lag far behind health and social programs for children and young adults. Consequently, the risk for abuse is higher for the elderly.[11] Hospitals, nursing homes, and rehabilitation and long-term care facilities place elders at high risk for abuse. In early studies abuse in long-term care facilities was examined. Pillemar and Moore[20] reported that 36% of employees they surveyed witnessed nursing home residents being physically abused, and 81% witnessed psychological abuse by employees in the past year. In a study done in Sweden, 11% of workers surveyed knew of at least one elder abuse incident in the past year.[21] Physical restraints, denial of dignity, deprivation of autonomy, and insufficient care are among the abusive acts against elders reported in institutions.[7]

COMMUNITY AWARENESS

Health care professionals, concerned citizens, and clear communication between professionals are crucial for the prevention of elder abuse, developing prevention initiatives, and identifying and reporting cases of suspected abuse. Raising community awareness through public education can be significant for preventing abuse and neglect. Education should include descriptions and examples of the many types of abuse, promoting community awareness and an understanding that abusive behavior in any form is not acceptable.[22]

Health care providers can be instrumental in screening, treating, educating, counseling, and referring elderly clients and their caregivers for appropriate services.[22] As with many health issue challenges experienced by the elderly, signs and symptoms of abuse are often overlooked by health professionals and are misconstrued to be the result of failing health and/or normal aging changes.[13,23,24] It is an alarming fact that fewer than 2% of reported cases of elder abuse come from health care providers and fewer than 10% include screening for abuse in their health examinations. Health care providers voice reasons for hesitancy in reporting suspected abuse as concerns of retaliation by the perpetrator on the health care provider or the victim of abuse, and being uncertain that they are not misinterpreting age-related physical and cognitive decline as abuse.[24] Health practitioners need to become more attentive to the different types of abuse, how to identify signs and symptoms of abuse, and know where victims of abuse can seek help.[24,25]

Law enforcement professionals are integral to protecting the elderly and enforcing laws that bring perpetrators to justice.[22] In cases of abuse police are often the first to respond, and their first responsibility is to ensure the safety of the victim. Police training programs should include topics on elder abuse and identify issues related to the unique needs of elderly citizens in their curricula. In addition, law enforcement procedures and policies need to be streamlined for reporting elder abuse and need to provide better access to services for elders when they cannot leave their homes.[26] An interdisciplinary approach that includes health care providers, social workers, law enforcement officials, and community agencies provides a means to screen, identify, intervene, and prevent further abuse.[2]

Community awareness initiatives that educate citizens about what constitutes abuse and neglect and what signs may indicate abuse can assist them in identifying abuse and in promptly reporting suspected abuse. Including topics of abuse in programs on successful aging and healthy living may be better received than discussing abuse in isolation of other aging issues. Such programs should identify services available to vulnerable elders in the community, county, and state, develop outreach programs that involve elders, friends, family, and community members, and advocate for better services and community involvement that are vital to addressing elder abuse.[2,26]

Family caregivers are poorly prepared to provide care to their elders, and may not know what community resources are available, when to use them, or how to access them. On average, caregivers caring for those 65 years or older are themselves older than 60 years old. One-third of these caregivers are also in fair to poor health.[27] Although caregivers may discuss the difficulties in their caregiving efforts, they are understandably reluctant to admit abuse.[2] Support groups, respite care, educational programs related to caring for the elderly, and financial planning for future elder care needs are all important for the wellbeing of caregivers and dependent elders.[28]

The media can take a more active role in discrediting negative stereotyping about aging and the elderly.[7,12,14,29] Attracting media attention about elder abuse is an effective tool in making the public aware of the issues of elder abuse, identifying resources, and gaining support to bring about community changes. At the same time policy makers will be educated about the issues of elder abuse and can make legislative changes that initiate effective services for elderly and their caregiver initiatives.[30,31]

SUMMARY

Elder abuse is a growing public health concern that affects elders regardless of their residence, socioeconomic status, or geographic locale. As "baby boomers" continue to age, the potential for elder abuse is likely to increase further impact on public health. Because there are few population-based studies, the magnitude of elder abuse is not fully realized. Personal, social, and cultural factors as they relate to the caregivers and the elders for whom they care influence prospects for elder abuse. Laws that protect the elderly are not standard, and definitions of elder abuse from nation to nation are inconsistent. Consequently, interventions for elder abuse are variable as well. Education about elder abuse should be a priority for everyone. Health care providers, social service workers, law enforcement officials, and communities should be educated about signs and symptoms, screening, identifying, reporting, and support services for the abused and abuser. Public policy changes are necessary to standardize and delineate guidelines and procedures for the prevention of elder abuse in the future.

REFERENCES

1. National Center on Elder Abuse. 15 questions & answers about elder abuse. Washington, DC: Author; 2005.
2. Patterson C. Canadian Task Force on the Periodic Health Examination. Periodic health examination, 1994 update: 4. Secondary prevention of elder abuse and mistreatment. CMAJ 1994;151:1413–20.
3. Dooley K, Schaffer D, Lance C, et al. Informal care can be better than adequate: development and evaluation of the exemplary care scale. Rehabil Psychol 2007; 52:359–69.
4. Elder justice now a national campaign to protect older Americans from abuse. 2009; Retrieved from: http://elderjusticenow.wordpress.com/2009/06/17/facts-about-elder-abuse-in-the-u-s/. Accessed February 22, 2011.
5. Sellas M. Elder abuse Medscape. 2011: Retrieved from: http://emedicine.medscape.com/article/805727-overview#a0199. Accessed February 22, 2011.
6. Cooper C, Selwood A, Livingston G. The prevalence of elder abuse and neglect: a systematic review. Age Ageing 2008;37:151–60.
7. World Health Organization. Missing voices: views of older persons on elder abuse. Geneva (Switzerland): World Health Organization; 2002. (WHO/NMH/VIP/02.1; WHO/NMH/NPH/02.2).
8. Bahugana N. Violence against elderly growing. Global action on aging. 2003; Retrieved from: http://www.globalaging.org/elderrights/world/violence.htm. Accessed January 12, 2011.
9. United Nations Elder Population Division. A global response to elder abuse and neglect. 2002; Retrieved from: www.un.org/esa/population/publications/worldageing19502050/pdf/90chapteriv.pdf. Accessed January 12, 2011.
10. National Institute of Justice. The national elder mistreatment study. Author. Washington, DC: National Institute of Justice; 2007.
11. Walsh C, Olson J, Ploeg J, et al. Elder abuse and oppression: voices of marginalized elders. J Elder Abuse Negl 2011;23:17–42.
12. Muehlbauer M, Crane P. Elder abuse and neglect. J Psychosoc Nurs 2006;44:43–8.
13. McGarry J, Simpson C. Identifying, reporting and preventing elder abuse in the practice setting. Nurs Older People 2008;21:33–8.
14. Stotkowski L. Forensic issues for nurses—elder abuse. Medscape. 2008; Retrieved from: http://cme.medscape.com/viewarticle/578859. Accessed February 22, 2011.
15. Acierno R, Hernandez-Tejada M, Muzzy W, et al. National elder mistreatment study final report. 2009; National Institute for Justice. Document 2226456. Retrieved from: http://www.ncjrs.gov/pdffiles1/nij/grants/226456.pdf. Accessed August 5, 2011.

16. American Psychological Association. Elder abuse: in search of solutions. 2011; Retrieved from: http://www.apa.org/pi/aging/resources/guides/elder-abuse.aspx. Accessed August 5, 2011.
17. Greenlee K. Taking a stand against elder abuse. 2011; Retrieved from: http://www.whitehouse.gov/blog/2011/06/13/taking-stand-against-elder-abuse. Accessed March 31, 2011.
18. Loue S. Elder abuse and neglect in medicine and law: the need for reform. J Leg Med 2001;22:159–201.
19. Otto J. Program and administrative issues affecting adult protective services. 2010; Public policy and aging report. Retrieved from: http://www.globalaging.org/elderrights/us/aps.htm. Accessed March 31, 2011.
20. Pillemar K, Moore D. Highlights from a study of abuse of patients in nursing homes. J Elder Abuse Negl 1990;2:5–29.
21. Saveman B, Astrom S, Bucht G, et al. Elder abuse in residential settings in Sweden. J Elder Abuse Negl 1999;10:43–60.
22. International Awareness of Elder Abuse. Elder abuse awareness community guide toolkit. Washington, DC: International Network for the Prevention of Elder Abuse; 2011.
23. Cronin G. Elder abuse: the same old story. Emerg Nurse 2007;15:11–3.
24. Perel-Levin S. Screening for elder abuse at the primary care level. Geneva (Switzerland): World Health Organization; 2008.
25. Bomba P. Use of a single page elder abuse assessment and management tool: a practical clinician's approach to identifying elder mistreatment. J Gerontol Soc Work 2009;46:102–23.
26. National Committee for the prevention of elder abuse. The role of professionals and concerned citizens. 2008. Retrieved from: http://www.preventelderabuse.org/elderabuse/professionals/. Accessed January 12, 2011.
27. Reinhard S, Given B, Petlick N, et al. Supporting family caregivers in providing care. In: Hughes R, editor. Patient safety and quality: an evidence-based handbook for nurses. Rockville (MD): Agency for Healthcare Research and Quality; 2008. Chapter 14.
28. National Center on Elder Abuse. Preventing elder abuse by family caregivers. Washington, DC: NCEA; 2009.
29. Weiland D. Abuse of older persons: an overview. Holist Nurs Pract 2000;14: 40–50.
30. Canadian Network for the Prevention of Elder Abuse. What role does media play in senior abuse prevention? 2010; Retrieved from: http://www.cnpea.ca/media_and_abuse__reporting.htm#Introduction. Accessed January 12, 2011.
31. Starr L. Preparing those caring for older adults to report elder abuse. J Contin Educ Nurs 2010;41:231–5.

The Relationship Between Abuse and Depression

Kelsey L. Hegarty, PhD

KEYWORDS

• Abuse • Intimate partner violence • Depression • Anxiety

Abuse is a very broad term (**Fig. 1**) and can include any abuse in relationships (eg, child, partner, elder, sibling) and other forms of violence against women (eg, sexual assault, genital mutilation). Depression also covers a range of diagnoses from depressive symptoms, minor depression, dysthymia, and major depression to bipolar disorder (**Box 1**). This article concentrates on intimate partner abuse and violence (IPA), also known as domestic or family violence, which is prevalent in communities globally.[1,2] The annual cost of IPA in Australia has been estimated at $13.2 billion, with similar figures in other countries.[3] The main cost to communities is from the mental health consequences of abuse, including depression, and depression is the single largest cause of disability burden in Australia.

IPA is defined as any behavior within an intimate relationship that causes physical, psychological, or sexual harm to those in the relationship.[4] This behavior includes acts of

- Physical violence (eg, pushed, hit, slapped, kicked, used knife or gun)
- Psychological abuse (eg, verbal abuse, humiliation, threats)
- Forced intercourse and other forms of sexual coercion, and
- Various controlling behaviors (eg, isolating from family and friends, monitoring movements, deprivation of basic necessities).

The World Health Organization (WHO) Multi-Country Study on women's health estimated that 15% to 71% of women had ever been physically or sexually assaulted by partners.[2] One in five ever-partnered women report physical or sexual abuse in a relationship.[1,5] Abuse is more common in clinical practice and estimates show that up to five women per week seen in general practices have experienced combined abuse at the hands of their partner.[6] Men are less likely than women to be victims of combined physical, emotional, and sexual abuse from their partners, and thus have been researched to a lesser extent.[5]

The author has nothing to disclose.

Department of General Practice, General Practice and Primary Health Care Academic Centre, University of Melbourne, 200 Berkeley Street, Carlton, Victoria 3068, Australia

E-mail address: k.hegarty@unimelb.edu.au

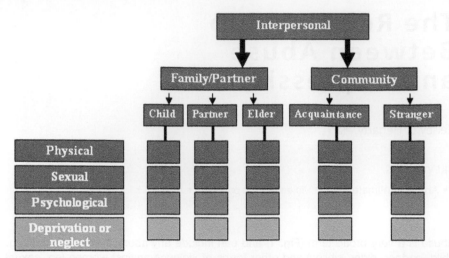

Fig. 1. Typology of violence. (*Adapted from* Krug EG, Mercy JA, Dahlberg LL, et al. The world report on violence and health. Lancet 2002;360(9339):1083–8; with permission.)

IPA is the leading contributor to death, disability, and illness in women of child-bearing age.[7] Most of this burden is from mental health issues, including depression.[8] Domestic violence has an intergenerational effect, with children who witness abuse having multiple health problems.[9] This article outlines the strong relationship that exists between abuse and depression. Although it focuses on intimate partner violence against women, it will also cover aspects of child abuse, perpetration of abuse, and depression.

Box 1
Depression glossary

Major depression

Clinical syndrome lasting 2 weeks with at least five of the following symptoms: depressed mood, loss of interest, significant weight loss or gain or appetite disturbance, insomnia or hypersomnia, psychomotor agitation or retardation, fatigue or loss of energy, feelings of worthlessness or excessive guilt, impaired thinking or concentration, indecisiveness, recurring thoughts of death, or suicidal thoughts.

Mild: mild disability, functions normally with effort

Moderate: no psychotic features, midway between mild and severe

Severe: most of the symptoms, observable disability with work or activities

Dysthymia

Chronic mild depressive disorder present on most days for 2 years with at least two of the following symptoms: appetite disturbance, insomnia or hypersomnia, decreased energy or fatigue, low self-esteem, decreased concentration or difficulty making decisions, or feelings of hopelessness.

Minor depression or subsyndromal depression

Acute mood disorder that is less severe than major depression lasting 2 weeks involving depressed mood or loss of interest with one to three of the major depression symptoms.

Data from APA. Diagnostic and statistical manual of mental disorders: DSM-IV. 4th edition. Washington, DC: American Psychiatric Association; 1994.

IPA RESULTS IN NEGATIVE MENTAL HEALTH OUTCOMES FOR WOMEN

Women experience depression approximately twice as often as men. The main reason for this, apart from women experiencing greater poverty, differing social roles, sex discrimination, and more negative life events, is that they experience a greater burden of violence and abuse.[10] The chronic stress and fear associated with living in an abusive relationship affects women's mental health in various ways.[11] A strong association exists between IPA and increased rates of anxiety, depression, alcohol and substance abuse, posttraumatic stress disorder (PTSD), and suicidality.[11] In a meta-analysis across 18 studies, the mean prevalence of depression among female victims of IPA was 47.6%, which is three to five times the prevalence reported among the general female population. Depression in abused women is associated with life stressors that accompany IPA, such as changes in residence, social isolation, marital separations, negative life events, low self-esteem, and child behavior problems.[12]

In clinical samples, the association is very strong.[13] For example, in a cross-sectional study of more than 1000 consecutive female patients attending general practice in Australia, 18.0% (218/1213) of women scored as currently probably depressed and 24.1% (277/1147) had experienced some type of abuse in an adult intimate relationship.[14] Depressed women were much more likely to have experienced some form of abuse (physical, emotional, or sexual) as a child (odds ratio [OR], 3.0, 95% CI, 2.1–4.2). Furthermore, depressed women were more likely to have experienced partner abuse, particularly severe combined abuse (OR, 8.0; 95% CI, 4.8–13.0), and physical and emotional abuse or harassment (OR, 8.1; 95% CI, 4.4–15.0). Even when these values were adjusted for all other variables, multidimensional measures of partner abuse remained highly associated with probable depression, with the magnitude of the effect being large.

When considering the association with depression, it is important to realize that across studies of abused women, the prevalence of PTSD is 63.8%, showing a considerable association between abuse and PTSD.[11] This mean prevalence is much greater than that seen in the general population of women,[11] with the experience of forced sex increasing PTSD symptoms almost threefold over physical violence alone.[15,16] Many women who have PTSD are often labeled by clinicians as having depression or bipolar disorder.[17] It is important for clinicians to screen for PTSD[18] if women are presenting with depressive or anxiety symptoms.

LINK WITH SUICIDE

Numerous studies also link suicidality to **interpersonal violence (IPV)** victimization, which includes actual deaths, self-harm, or suicidal gestures, attempts, ideation, or threats. Investigators have suggested that with ongoing abuse, the suicidality progresses in severity and lethality over time. The WHO Multi-Country Study reported that approximately 10% of IPV victims reported suicidal behaviors in their lifetime.[2]

THEORIES REGARDING THE LINK BETWEEN IPV AND DEPRESSION

Many theories exist as to why abuse and depression are associated. One explanation is that multiple or ongoing victimization increases women's vulnerability to depression. Women who experience victimization in childhood and as adults are more likely to experience depression and PTSD as an adult.[13,19] In support of this, a recent systematic review found that domestic violence was a consistent factor that predicted antenatal depression.[20] Other feminist explanations suggest that women who are depressed and have low self-esteem are less likely to be able to escape the violence and abuse. A further hypothesis suggests that relationship power accounts for some of the association between intimate partner violence and depression. In one study, women who felt powerless had higher rates of IPA and higher levels of depression, with a mediation analysis showing that sexual relationship power mediated the relationship between intimate partner violence and depression.[21]

In contrast to this, several United States studies have examined whether depression during adolescence predicts later victimization. In a community sample of 610 young adults,[22] youth history of depression by 15 years of age predicted victimization at 20 years of age. Results from a school sample of 1659 young women also suggest that depressive symptoms among girls during adolescence are associated with increased risk of subsequent exposure to physical partner violence. These results could be confounded by a history of child abuse, which could result in depression and make the subsequent revictimization more likely.[23]

Alcohol and drug use is another mental health outcome frequently seen among victims of IPA that plays a role in the association between abuse and depression.[24] Investigators have suggested that substance use is an outcome of IPV through PTSD, and that the relationship between substance abuse and IPA is cyclical in nature.[25] For example, childhood abuse and all forms of violence are causes of PTSD and substance use, although in turn substance use can also be seen as a risk factor for further violence and abuse. Self-report data have shown that substance abuse increases after physical assault, sexual abuse, or a traumatic event. The risk of developing a substance abuse problem involving alcohol is stronger than for drugs after experiencing IPV.[25]

Finally, the issue of poverty has been raised,[26] whereby both poverty and IPA result in PTSD, social isolation, and depression, and financial matters must be addressed when examining the link between IPA and depression. The ecological model of causation of IPA outlined by the WHO is a broad theoretical model incorporating many of the factors discussed earlier (**Fig. 2**).

NATURE OF THE ASSOCIATION OVER TIME

Although some women have chronic depression that is exacerbated by the abusive relationship, prevalence of depression decreases as women gain temporal distance from victimization. If the abuse stops in a relationship, then women's scores on depression measures decrease.[27] If the abuse is ongoing then depression scores increase.[28] The fact that high rates of depression are seen for more than one form of violence suggests that abuse causes the depression.[29,30] Similarly, help-seeking and safety behaviors, including disclosure, counseling, intervention orders, and stopping the violence, significantly decrease depression and PTSD symptoms.[16]

In one clinical study,[13] IPA had the strongest associations (more than child abuse) with mental health problems, increased for experiences in the past year (anxiety: OR, 3.3; 95% CI 2.2–4.8; depression: OR, 2.7; 95% CI, 1.4–5.4; PTSD: OR, 3.2; 95% CI, 1.7–6.1; and suicide attempt: OR, 2.1; 95% CI, 1.2–3.7).

PERPETRATORS OF IPV

Investigation into the link between perpetration of IPA and depression has been limited. In a prevalence study from general practice, 13.5% of men used abusive behavior in the past 12 months. Depression, alcohol use, and personal history of abuse were the most important predictors of using abuse and violence toward a partner.[31] Similarly, in a qualitative study from general practice, depression, stress,

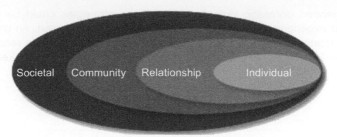

Fig. 2. Ecological model. Individual: the first level identifies biologic and personal history factors that increase the likelihood of becoming a victim or perpetrator of violence, including age, education, income, substance use, and history of abuse. Relationship: the second level includes factors that increase risk because of relationships with peers, intimate partners, and family members. The closest social circle (peers, partners, and family members) influences behavior and contributes to a person's range of experience. Community: the third level explores the settings, such as schools, workplaces, and neighborhoods, in which social relationships occur, and seeks to identify the characteristics of these settings that are associated with becoming victims or perpetrators of violence. Societal: the fourth level examines the broad societal factors that help create a climate in which violence is encouraged or inhibited, including social and cultural norms. Other large societal factors include the health, economic, educational, and social policies that help to maintain economic or social inequalities between groups in society. (*From* Dahlberg LL, Krug EG. Violence-a global public health problem. In: Krug E, Dahlberg LL, Mercy JA, et al, editors. World Report on Violence and Health. Geneva (Switzerland): World Health Organization; 2002. p. 1–56; with permission.)

suicidal ideation, alcohol or drug abuse, anger problems, relationship problems, and recent separation were the main presentations in men who used violence in their relationship.[32] However, men may also be the victims of abuse at the hands of their female partners, and depression may play a role in this violence.

INTERVENING TO REDUCE THE ASSOCIATION BETWEEN IPV AND DEPRESSION

Increasing abused women's safety and reducing exposure to violence are key to minimizing negative mental health consequences for women. Despite the strong association, information and advice for nurses working in clinical settings are lacking. Nurses who work in antenatal, emergency, family practice, mental health, and drug services must be equipped to recognize and respond to IPA and the sequelae of child abuse. Many barriers exist to inquiry by health professionals[33–35] and disclosure by patients.[14] This lack of discussion has inspired a movement, particularly in the United States, toward screening of all women in clinical settings. A recent Cochrane review, however, stated that no current evidence supports this move.[36] Nurses have been at the forefront of the call for action in the area of abuse. However, the evidence supporting action is greatly lacking. Currently, investigators suggest that routine inquiry would be useful if nurses feel equipped to respond to women in clinical practice.[36] What is known, however, is that when women present with depression, anxiety, insomnia, suicidal ideation, and PTSD, they likely have underlying abuse and violence issues.

Nurses should respond to abused women using advocacy, empowerment, and safety-based interventions.[37] These methods have been shown to provide some benefits for women.[36] Group and individual psychological therapies provided by trained mental health nurses are also likely to reduce depression in women who have experienced domestic violence. All of these strategies could be offered to women who experience the dual diagnosis of IPA and depression. An urgent need exists to educate nurses and implement systems to support them in responding to women experiencing abuse and violence. The hope is that this will then keep women and children safe.

REFERENCES

1. Australian Bureau of Statistics. Personal Safety Survey, 2005. Available at: http://www.ausstats.abs.gov.au/ausstats/subscriber.nsf/0/056A404DAA576AE6CA2571D00080E985/$File/49060_2005%20(reissue).pdf. Accessed August 23, 2011.
2. World Health Organization. WHO Multi-Country Study on women's health and domestic violence against women: summary report of initial results on prevalence, health outcomes and women's responses. Geneva (Switzerland): WHO; 2005.
3. Access Economics. The cost of domestic violence to the Australian economy: Part 1 2004. Available at: http://www.fahcsia.gov.au/sa/women/pubs/violence/cost_violence_economy_2004/Documents/cost_of_dv_to_australian_economy_i.pdf. Accessed August 23, 2011.
4. Krug EG, Mercy JA, Dahlberg LL, et al. The world report on violence and health. Lancet 2002;360(9339):1083–8.
5. Tjaden P, Thoennes N. Extent, nature, and consequences of intimate partner violence. Washington, DC: U.S. Department of Justice; 2000.
6. Hegarty K. What is domestic violence and how common is it? In: Roberts G, Hegarty K, Feder G, editors. Intimate partner abuse and health professionals: new approaches to domestic violence. London: Elsevier; 2006. p. 18–29.
7. The health costs of violence. Measuring the burden of diseases caused by intimate partner violence. Melbourne (Australia): VicHealth; 2005.
8. Campbell JC. Health consequences of intimate partner violence. Lancet 2002; 359:1331–6.
9. Bedi G, Goddard C. Intimate partner violence: what are the impacts on children? Aust Psychol 2007;42(1):66–77.
10. Astbury J, Cabral M. Women's mental health: an evidence based review. Geneva (Switzerland): World Health Organisation; 2000.
11. Golding J. Intimate partner violence as a risk factor for mental disorders: a meta-analysis. J Fam Violence 1999;14(2):99–132.
12. Dienemann J, Boyle E, Baker D, et al. Intimate partner abuse among women diagnosed with depression. Issues Ment Health Nurs 2000;21(5):499–513.
13. Coid J, Petruckevitch A, Chung WS, et al. Abusive experiences and psychiatric morbidity in women primary care attenders. Br J Psychiatry 2003;183:332–9 [discussion: 40–1].
14. Hegarty K, Gunn J, Chondros P, et al. Association between depression and abuse by partners of women attending general practice: descriptive, cross sectional survey. BMJ 2004;328(7440):621–4.
15. Campbell J, Kub L, Nedd D. Voices of strength and resistance: a contextual and longitudinal analysis of women's responses to battering. J Interpers Violence 1998;13:743–62.
16. Coker AL, Weston R, Creson DL, et al. PTSD symptoms among men and women survivors of intimate partner violence: the role of risk and protective factors. Violence Vict 2005;20(6):625–43.

17. Campbell J, Laughon K, Woods A. Impact of intimate partner abuse on physical and mental health: how does it present in clinical practice? In: Roberts G, Hegarty K, Feder G, editors. Intimate partner abuse and health professionals: new approaches to domestic violence. London: Elsevier; 2006. p. 43–60.
18. Blanchard EB, Jones-Alexander J, Buckley TC, et al. Psychometric properties of the PTSD Checklist (PCL). Behav Res Ther 1996;34(8):669–73.
19. Roberts SJ, Sorensen L. Prevalence of childhood sexual abuse and related sequelae in a lesbian population. J Gay Lesb Med Assoc 1999;3(1):11–9.
20. Lancaster CA, Gold KJ, Flynn HA, et al. Risk factors for depressive symptoms during pregnancy: a systematic review. Am J Obstet Gynecol 2010;202(1):5–14.
21. Filson J, Ulloa E, Runfola C, et al. Does powerlessness explain the relationship between intimate partner violence and depression? J Interpers Violence 2010; 25(3):400–15.
22. Keenan-Miller D, Hammen C, Brennan P. Adolescent psychosocial risk factors for severe intimate partner violence in young adulthood. J Consult Clin Psychol 2007; 75(3):456–63.
23. Wekerle C, Leung E, Wall AM, et al. The contribution of childhood emotional abuse to teen dating violence among child protective services-involved youth. Child Abuse Negl 2009;33(1):45–58.
24. Gilchrist G, Hegarty K, Chondros P, et al. The association between intimate partner violence, alcohol and depression in family practice. BMC Fam Pract 2010;11:72–8.
25. Kilpatrick DG, Acierno R, Resnick HS, et al. A two-year longitudinal analysis of the relationships between violent assault and substance use in women. J Consult Clin Psychol 1997;65(5):4–47.
26. Goodman LA, Smyth KF, Borges AM, et al. When crises collide: how intimate partner violence and poverty intersect to shape women's mental health and coping? Trauma Violence Abuse 2009;10(4):306–29.
27. Campbell JC. Helping women understand their risk in situations of intimate partner violence. J Interpers Violence 2004;19(12):1464–77.
28. Sutherland C, Bybee D, Sullivan C. The long-term effects of battering on women's health. Womens Health 1998;4(1):41–70.
29. Mullen P, Romans-Clarkson S, Walton V, et al. Impact of sexual and physical abuse on women's mental health. Lancet 1988;1(8590):841–5.
30. Roberts GL, Williams GM, Lawrence JM, et al. How does domestic violence affect women's mental health? Women Health 1998;28(1):117–29.
31. Oriel MF. Screening men for partner violence in a primary care setting. A new strategy for detecting domestic violence. J Fam Pract 1998;46(6):493–8.
32. Taft A, Broom DH, Legge D. General practitioner management of intimate partner abuse and the whole family: qualitative study. BMJ 2004;328(7440):618.
33. Hegarty K, Feder G, Ramsay J. Identification of partner abuse in health care settings: should health professionals be screening? In: Roberts G, Hegarty K, Feder G, editors. Intimate partner abuse and health professionals. London: Elsevier; 2006. p. 45–58.
34. Rose D, Trevillion K, Woodall A, et al. Barriers and facilitators of disclosures of domestic violence by mental health service users: qualitative study. Br J Psychiatry 2011;198:189–94.
35. Bacchus L, Mezey G, Bewley S, et al. Prevalence of domestic violence when midwives routinely enquire in pregnancy. BJOG 2004;111(5):441–5.
36. Feder G, Ramsay J, Dunne D, et al. How far does screening women for domestic (partner) violence in different health-care settings meet criteria for a screening

programme? Systematic reviews of nine UK National Screening Committee criteria. Health Technol Assess 2009;13(16):iii–iv, xi–xiii, 1–113, 37–347.

37. Ramsay J, Carter Y, Davidson L, et al. Advocacy interventions to reduce or eliminate violence and promote the physical and psychosocial well-being of women who experience intimate partner abuse. Cochrane Database Syst Rev 2009;3: CD005043.

Family Issues Associated with Military Deployment, Family Violence, and Military Sexual Trauma

Cira Fraser, PhD, RN, ACNS-BC*

KEYWORDS

• Military • Deployment • Family • Military sexual trauma
• Violence • Abuse • Neglect

The United States military has been in involved in conflicts in Iraq and Afghanistan for a decade. There is increasing interest in and concern for the effects of deployment on service members and their families.[1] Emerging research suggests that the health effects of deployment are significant.[2] The effect of deployment on families is complex and needs to be better understood.[1] There is a paucity of research on military deployment and its effects on military families.[3]

Today's military has a greater percentage of families and children in comparison with previous generations. There are many and unique demands on military families made by the ongoing conflicts.[1] Military life can be stressful.[4] The pile-up of life changes (the sum of normative, nonnormative, and intrafamily strains) may have negative consequences in the family system and/or its members.[5,6] The presence of an increasing number of stressors is associated with an increased likelihood of domestic violence in veterans.[7] Military sexual trauma may be experienced by some service members during both deployment and assignments at duty stations. It is a psychological trauma resulting from physical assault of a sexual nature, battery of a sexual nature, or sexual harassment. Sexual trauma is associated with several negative psychological and physical outcomes.[8]

The author has nothing to disclose.
Monmouth University, Marjorie K. Unterberg School of Nursing and Health Studies, 400 Cedar Avenue, West Long Branch, NJ 07764-1898, USA
* 44 Wiman Avenue, Staten Island, NY 10308.
E-mail addresses: cfraser@monmouth.edu; cirafraser@si.rr.com

Nurs Clin N Am 46 (2011) 445–455
doi:10.1016/j.cnur.2011.08.011
0029-6465/11/$ – see front matter © 2011 Elsevier Inc. All rights reserved.

In this article, literature and research are presented to provide an overview of military deployment and families, and the effect of deployment on families; this is followed by a review of research on family violence and military sexual trauma.

MILITARY DEPLOYMENT AND FAMILIES

Military deployment can be conceptualized in several different ways.[1] The purpose of deployments may be for training, peacekeeping, or combat. The level of danger and risk varies based on the type of deployment. The amount of notice prior to deployment may also vary. The length of time of deployment can typically range from 6 to 18 months. Deployment can also be conceptualized as a process that begins long before the service member leaves and continues beyond his or her return home. Sheppard and colleagues[1] propose a model of the effect of the deployment process on family stability, with the predeployment and postdeployment periods as being most challenging for family stability. The predeployment and postdeployment periods are most disruptive due to the increased challenges and family stress, whereas during the actual time the service member is deployed, family stability may even be higher than baseline for the family.

Predeployment, the deployment phase and resilience, and return from deployment can have an impact on family functioning.[9] Predeployment can take up to 6 months to a year, and may involve training, testing, and practicing for the mission. Notification of deployment can be stressful for the family. Other stressors may include pregnancy; an illness of a child, spouse, or parent; dealing with marital problems or interruption of a planned marriage, separation, or divorce; an interruption of education; and missing key milestones of family members. Planning for deployment may place many demands on the family. Decisions may involve where the family will live during the deployment (stay in the military housing or move closer to family). There is updating of wills, power of attorney, and other legal documents. Arrangements are made for home maintenance, paying bills, and a shifting of tasks to the nondeploying partner. Preparations are made to maintain communication between the deploying family member and children and family. Other preparations may include the deploying parent leaving keepsakes for the children, such as photos and maps showing where they will be while deployed. Stressors may also result from the uncertainty of exactly where the family member will be deployed and how much of a threat the type of deployment may pose.[9]

Stressors for the family during the deployment phase may include the actual departure of the deployed family member, dealing with the absence of the family member, loneliness, and the fears related to the deployed member's safety and well-being. Communication via cell phone, email, webcams, and photos may be welcome, but can also serve as a source of stress.[9]

About 1 month before the return from deployment, the deployed member and family may experience optimistic expectations for a family reunion. However, the actual return of the deployed member may result in numerous stressors attributable to the changes that may have occurred during the deployment period. Changes may include, but are not limited to, new routines of the nondeployed family member and children; financial issues; and changes in roles, relationships, and expectations. The deployed family member may have experienced combat exposure resulting in posttraumatic stress disorder (PTSD).[9] Military children appear to be at greater risk of abuse related to parenting skills, negative parent-child interactions, and hostility and violence following combat during deployment. Child abuse is more common in enlisted service members.[4] The numerous stressors faced before, during, and following deployment can all have a negative impact on the family.

RESEARCH ON THE EFFECT OF DEPLOYMENT ON FAMILIES

Intimate partner violence in the deploying military was investigated by Fonseca and colleagues,[10] who examined whether alcohol use, stress, demographics, and relationship satisfaction predicted intimate partner violence in soldiers preparing for deployment. The sample included 2926 participants who reported being married or living with a partner. The instruments used were a demographic questionnaire, the CAGE questionnaire to assess problematic alcohol-related behaviors, a single item on the Dyadic Adjustment Scale to measure relationship satisfaction, 5 questions on the Health Enrollment Assessment Review that measures stress, and the Conflict Tactics Scale that assesses the range of tactics (from calm discussion to use of a knife or gun) used when dealing with disagreements with their intimate partner. Of the 2926 participants, 449 were identified as engaging in intimate partner violence within the past year. The prevalence of intimate partner violence was found to be 15.8% in this study, reported as similar to previous research in nondeploying participants. The 5 significant predictors of self-reported intimate partner violence were younger age, less education, more stress, less relationship satisfaction, and risky alcohol behaviors. There was a nearly double increase in the likelihood of intimate partner violence associated with risky alcohol behaviors.

Warner and colleagues[11] investigated the psychological effects of deployment on 295 spouses of military service members at the time of departure. The effects of demographic factors, prior deployments, and stress on depressive symptoms were examined. The majority of the sample was female (96.3%), white (79.7%), married to an enlisted military service member (86.1%), and with some college education or a college degree (74.2%). The 5 most frequently reported deployment stressors were found to be the safety of the deployed spouse (96.3%), feeling lonely (89.8%), raising a young child alone (63.1%), having problems communicating with the deployed spouse (64.4%), and caring/raising/disciplining children when spouse is deployed spouse (56.3%). Forty-three percent of the participants had moderate or severe depressive symptoms. Each increased point on the Perceived Stress Scale was associated with a 1.21-times greater risk of depression as measured by the Patient Health Questionnaire 9.

The effect of deployment on young children was investigated by Barker and Berry.[12] The sample included 57 families who had at least one young child under the age of 4 years. Twenty-one families made up the single deployment group, the multiple deployment group included 22 families, and the nondeployment group included 14 families. There were two data collection times; the first, 3 to 4 months into the parents' deployment and the second, approximately 4 to 6 weeks after the parent returned home from deployment. The first survey asked basic demographic questions, with a retrospective rating of the child's intense attachment behaviors and observed behavior responses. The questions were developed by the investigators. The second survey requested information about events during the deployment, assessed to rate the child's intense attachment behaviors and observed behavior responses for the reunion. Children with a deployed parent had increased behavior problems when the parent was deployed and increased attachment behaviors on the parents' return. Children described as "difficult" were found to be more likely to have behavioral problems during deployment. Older toddlers and preschoolers were found to be more prone than infants to behavioral problems. The problem behaviors during deployment included the following: needs lots of attention (57.5%), clinginess (42.5%), increased temper tantrums (42.5%), asking lots of questions about the deployed parent (37.5%), wants to control things (37.5%), defiant/disobedient (32.5%), argues/fights (25%), appetite changes (22.5%), prolonged crying (22.5%), and sleeping problems/nightmares (20%). Problem behaviors occurring on the return of the deployed parent were found to include: not wanting to sleep in own bed (40%), preferred nondeployed parent or caregiver (37.5%), did not want returning parent to leave room or house (37.5%), ignored returning parent (22.5%), and did not let returning parent comfort him/her (22.5%).

The effect of deployment on adolescents was investigated by Huebner and colleagues.[13] Focus groups were used with adolescents to explore uncertainty, loss, resilience, and adjustment when a parent was deployed. The focus groups were held in 5 states and included a sample of 107 participants who ranged in age from 12 to 18 years. Most of the adolescents' parents were deployed to Iraq or Afghanistan. Fifty-four percent were boys and 46% were girls. The transcripts from the focus groups were analyzed using the constant comparative method. The adolescents experienced a range of emotions related to the deployment of the parent. Behavioral changes included a tendency for emotional outbursts and acting out toward others. Depression and anxiety were found to be common. The participants during the deployment process were required to assume roles and responsibilities, then relinquish them. The return of the deployed parent was found to be more difficult than the absence of the parent. The effect of deployment on the family system included conflict and uncontrolled "lashing out" with the nondeployed parent, who most often was the mother. It was perceived that the parent had a shorter temper, was under stressed, and had signs of depression. These changes had a negative effect on the relationship between the nondeployed parent and the adolescent. The participants also experienced difficulty when the parent returning from deployment failed to acknowledge changes and thought everything should be the same as before he or she left. The returning parent also failed to recognize or appreciate that the adolescent had matured during the deployment.

FAMILY VIOLENCE IN MILITARY FAMILIES

Rentz and colleagues[3] state that family violence in the military may be higher than in civilian families because of the higher stress levels related to the military lifestyle. In their review of the literature on family violence in the military the investigators found few studies. There were even fewer studies comparing family violence in military and civilian families. The most common form of child maltreatment was physical abuse, ranging from 31.3% to 70.8% of all child maltreatment cases. Child neglect was also found to be a common problem in military families, accounting for 18.5% to 50.0% of child maltreatment studies found in the literature. Sexual abuse was the least common, accounting for 6.1% to 17.8%, with emotional abuse of children accounting for 0.7% to 15.6% of child maltreatment. For spouses, physical abuse was most common in military families. Studies the investigators were able to find that compared military and civilian families showed mixed results. Some studies reported greater family violence in the military whereas others indicated that family violence was lower in the military families.

The trends in child maltreatment in Army families were examined by McCarroll and colleagues.[14] The time span covered was 1990 to 2004. Data from the Army Central Registry were examined. Ninety percent of those involved in the child maltreatment cases were the parents of the child. Fifty-six percent were fathers and 44% were mothers. The average age of the parents was 29 years. The investigators found that from 1990 to 2004 there was an overall decrease in the rate of child maltreatment in the United States Army. This finding was mainly attributable to the decrease in child physical abuse. Also, the rate of sexual abuse decreased a small amount. Emotional abuse showed fluctuations, with a small increase reflected between 2000 and 2004. During the period 1990 to 2004 the neglect rate increased about 41% and reached its highest level in 2004. The highest rate of neglect was for children younger than 1 year. The investigators compared the rates in Army families with the United States national figures, and concluded that the trend in the Army families was similar to that of the general population.

Predictors of child abuse in Army families were investigated by Schaeffer and colleagues.[15] The investigators pointed out the paucity of research comparing predictors for mother and fathers separately. The participants included 590 mothers and 175 fathers from 27 Army installations in the United States, Germany, and Japan. Most of the active-duty family members were the fathers (93%). Most of the participants lived off-base in civilian housing. Forty-seven percent lived on base. The average age of participants was 24.4 years for the mothers and 26.4 years for the fathers. Six self-report instruments were used to determine child abuse potential: the Center for Epidemiologic Studies Depression Scale, the Child Abuse Potential Inventory, the Abuse Subscale, the Family Environment Scale, Real Form to measure perception of family functioning, the revised Dyadic Adjustment Scale to assess how happy people are with a romantic partner, the Parenting Stress Index, Short Form, and Social Support Questionnaire, 6-item version. The significant predictors of child abuse potential for mothers were depression, parental stress, family conflict, family cohesion, marital adjustment, and satisfaction with social support. For fathers there were 4 significant predictors of child abuse potential: depression, parental stress, family conflict, and family expressiveness.

Forgey and Badger[16] investigated patterns of intimate partner violence in married women in the military. The sample included 248 enlisted women in the Army who were married to civilian spouses. The mean age of the participants was 29.8 years and the mean age for spouses was 31.8 years. Ethnicity was as follows: black 40%, white 37%, Hispanic 11%, Asian Pacific 5%, Native American 3%, and others 4%. The mean length of time in the service was 7.1 years. The mean number of years married was 6.2 years. The education level of the military women was high school diploma 52%, associate degree 35%, and bachelor degree or higher 7.3%. The education levels of the spouses were GED or high school diploma 76%, associate degree 17%, and bachelor or graduate degree 5.6%. The instruments used to collect data were a demographic questionnaire and the Conflict Tactics Scale 2. The investigators found that the sample of women enlisted in the Army were almost 4 times more likely to be victims of unilateral violence from their nonmilitary spouses than to be perpetrators of unilateral violence. The women were also 3 times more likely to be victims of severe violence from their spouses. Moreover, the women were twice as likely to be involved in asymmetric bidirectional violence whereby the spouse was inflicting a higher level of violence. The investigators state that the findings of this study are similar to nonmilitary studies of intimate partner violence.

MILITARY SEXUAL TRAUMA

The definition of military sexual trauma used by the Department of Veterans Affairs (VA) is given by US Code (1720D of Title 38). It is "psychological trauma, which in the judgment of a VA mental health professional, resulted from a physical assault of a sexual nature, battery of a sexual nature, or sexual harassment which occurred while the veteran was serving on active duty or active duty for training." Sexual harassment is further defined as "repeated, unsolicited verbal or physical contact of a sexual nature which is threatening in character." (US Department of Veterans Affairs, 2010).

Suras and Lind[17] reviewed the literature on military sexual assault, and state that risk factors for military sexual trauma are associated with being an enlisted service member who entered the military at a younger age and being less likely to have completed college. The prevalence rate is estimated to be between 17% and 30% when mailed or telephone surveys are used. The mental health consequences of military sexual trauma evident in the literature include psychological symptoms, such as depression and alcohol abuse, and an association with an increased likelihood of PTSD. Women veterans with a history of military sexual trauma are 9 times more likely to develop PTSD than women with no history of sexual assault. The physical health consequences of military sexual trauma evident in the literature include current physical symptoms (menstrual problems, pelvic pain, back pain, headaches, gastrointestinal symptoms, and chronic fatigue) and increased cardiovascular risk factors (obesity, smoking, and sedentary lifestyles).

The effect of sexual stressors on functioning and psychiatric symptoms in active-duty military men and women was investigated by Murdoch and colleagues.[18] Sexual stressors included sexual identity challenges, sexual harassment, and sexual assault. The sample included 487 men and 327 women stationed in the United States. The mean age for the men was 34 years and for the women 34.2 years. Twenty-five percent of the men reported at least one sexual identity challenge, 36% had at least one sexual harassment experience, and 1.2% experienced sexual assault. Forty percent of women reported at least one sexual identity challenge, 78% experienced at least one sexual harassment episode, and 10.5% experienced sexual assault. Participants who reported more types of sexual stressors had more depression and anxiety, and more severe PTSD and somatic complaints when compared with those who had fewer or no sexual stressors.

Street and colleagues[19] examined the prevalence of sexual harassment and sexual assault as well as health outcomes in former reservists who completed military service by the year 2000. The average length of time in service was 9.1 years. The sample included 2318 women and 1628 men representing the Army, Navy, Marine, Air Force, and Coast Guard Reserves. The data were collected using the Sexual Experiences Questionnaire, Center for Epidemiologic Studies Depression Scale, the PTSD Checklist, and a somatic symptoms measure developed by the investigators to measure pain, gastrointestinal symptoms, psychoneurologic symptoms, sexual symptoms, menstrual symptoms (women) and sexual dysfunction (men). Approximately 60% of the women had a history of sexual harassment and 13.1% reported being sexually assaulted. The women who experienced sexual harassment or sexual assault were more likely to be between 30 and 49 years of age, white, highly educated, served in the reserves more than 5 years, and more likely to have a service-related disability. Approximately 27% of the men had a history of sexual harassment and 1.6% reported being sexually assaulted. The men who experienced sexual harassment or sexual assault were similar in demographics to the other men in the study. The findings revealed that for women, reports of sexual harassment were associated with greater risk of somatic symptoms, depression, and medical conditions. When both sexual harassment and sexual assault were experienced, the risk of somatic symptoms, depression, and medical conditions was even greater. For men who experienced sexual harassment there was a greater risk of somatic symptoms, depression, and medical conditions. When both sexual harassment and sexual assault were experienced, there was a strong association with depression and somatic symptoms.

The Veterans Health Administration screening program for military sexual violence was examined by Kimerling and colleagues.[20] Data for 185,880 women and 4,139,888 men who were treated in the VA health care settings was examined. The majority of patients (70%) had been screened for military sexual trauma. Those that screened positive had greater odds of having mental health comorbidities, including PTSD. These patients also had greater odds of having medical comorbidities (liver disease, chronic pulmonary disease and, for women, weight conditions). Some gender differences emerged. PTSD had the strongest association with military sexual trauma and was 3 times stronger for women when compared with male veterans. Alcohol disorders and anxiety disorders were more common for both male and female veterans, but the relationship was stronger among women. In women, obesity, weight loss, and hypothyroidism were associated with military sexual trauma. In men, AIDS was more common in men who reported military sexual trauma.

There is a growing number of women veterans who served in Afghanistan and Iraq and who are now seeking the care provided by the VA. Haskell and colleagues[21] conducted a retrospective study to determine the prevalence of military sexual trauma, PTSD, pain, obesity, and depression in veterans receiving care from the VA in Connecticut. The sample included 1032 men and 197 women who received care between 2001 and 2007. Approximately 90% were screened for military sexual trauma, PTSD, and depression. The investigators found that more women screened positive for military sexual trauma (14%) and depression (48%) compared with men (1% and 39%, respectively). More men screened positive for PTSD (33%), pain (45%), and obesity (21%) compared with women (21%, 38%, and 13%, respectively).

Military sexual trauma, problematic health behaviors, and psychological distress in 232 female veterans seeking care for mental health issues was investigated by Rowe and colleagues.[22] The mean age of participants was 44.9 years with 76.1% being Caucasian, 15.3% African American, 5.5% Hispanic, and 12.8% other. The instruments used included the Survey of Health Behaviors, Beck Depression Inventory, Trauma Symptom Inventory, and VA MST Screen to assess military sexual trauma. Approximately two-thirds of the sample reported experiencing military sexual trauma. These women were more likely to engage in starving behavior and to self-identify as disabled, and had more severe symptoms and functional impairment associated with physical or emotional injury when compared with women who had not experienced military sexual trauma.

The relationship between sexual assault and gynecologic symptoms was investigated by Campbell and colleagues.[23] The sample included 298 women recruited from a women's VA clinic. The majority were veterans and African American. The instruments used for data collection were the Sexual Experiences Survey, a questionnaire on assault characteristics, and 6 items from the Cohen-Hoberman Inventory of Physical Symptoms and a sociodemographic questionnaire. The findings revealed that the rate of lifetime sexual assault for this sample was 37%. At least 14% of the total sample was sexually assaulted during service in the military. The participants with a history of sexual assault (n = 134) experienced significantly more frequency of symptoms of pelvic pain, vaginal bleeding/discharge, painful intercourse, rectal bleeding, bladder infections, and painful urination when compared with those who were not sexually assaulted.

The relationship between suicide attempts in the military and the relationship with traumatic events was investigated by Belik and colleagues.[24] The sample included 5049 men and 2077 women who were Canadian military personnel, ranging in age from 16 to 54 years. The response rate was 81.1%. Suicide attempts were reported by 2.2% of the men and 5.6% of the women. Interpersonal traumas and sexual assault were found to be associated with suicide attempts. For men the odds ratio ranged from 2.31 to 4.43 and for women the odds ratio ranged from 1.73 to 3.71. The investigators also found that the number of traumatic events was associated with an increased risk of suicide in this sample. The investigators concluded that this study was the first to show that sexual and other traumatic events were significantly associated with an increased risk of suicide in military men and women.

McCall-Hosenfeld and colleagues[25] investigated mediators of sexual assault in the military and decreased sexual satisfaction. The 4 mediators tested were physical health-related quality of life, emotional health-related quality of life, gynecologic illness, and lack of a close partner. The sample included a national survey of 3632 women veterans who used VA outpatient services. The demographics were categorized based on participant-reported sexual satisfaction. Those who reported being sexually satisfied were a mean age of 46 years with ethnicity reported as white (75%), black (19%), and other (6%). Marital status was married/partnered (45%), divorced/separated (29%), widowed (8%), and never married (19%). Those who reported being sexually dissatisfied were a mean age of 43 years with ethnicity reported as white (72%), black (21%), and other (7%). Marital status was married/partnered (33%), divorced/separated (39%), widowed (6%), and never married (21%). Participants who were sexually dissatisfied were found to be more likely to endorse alcohol abuse and smoking. Of the 3632 participants, 24% reported a history of sexual assault in the military. Increased physical health-related quality of life, having a close partner, and lack of gynecologic morbidity mediated the adverse sexual assault in the military and sexual satisfaction. A decreased mental health-related quality of life was found to mediate the association between sexual assault in the military and sexual dissatisfaction.

SUMMARY

Numerous stressors related to military life and the deployment process can pile up and overwhelm the family's ability to cope effectively. Along with dealing with multiple stressors, the service members returning from combat areas may experience PTSD, further affecting family functioning. Conflict, violence, and abuse may occur in some service members and military families. A review of the literature revealed that some research has been done with military families, but much more needs to be done especially because of the increase in deployments to combat areas since 2001. The research presented in this article provides an overview of the issues investigated in recent years.

Research on the effect of deployment on families revealed that significant predictors of intimate partner violence in deploying service members were younger age, less education, more stress, less relationship satisfaction, and risky alcohol behaviors. The risky alcohol behaviors nearly doubled the likelihood of intimate partner violence. Stressors most frequently reported by spouses of military service members at the time of departure were found to be concern for the safety of the deploying spouse, feeling lonely, raising a young child alone, having problems communicating with spouse deployed, and caring/raising/disciplining children. Increased stress was found to be associated with a greater risk for depression.

The effect of deployment on children younger than 4 was found to be associated with problem behaviors that included increased temper tantrums, defiant/disobedient behavior, arguments and fights, a preference for the nondeployed parent, ignoring the returning parent, not allowing the returning parent to comfort him or her, and several other behaviors. Adolescents aged 12 to 18 were also found to have behavioral changes that included a tendency for emotional outbursts, acting out toward others, conflict, uncontrolled "lashing out," difficulty relating to the parent returning from deployment, among several other behaviors.

Reviews of the literature have stated that the most common form of child maltreatment is physical abuse and neglect. The least common was found to be sexual abuse. For spouses, physical abuse was most common. Comparisons of military and civilian families were mixed, with some finding greater family violence in the military but others finding the opposite. An examination of trends by one study revealed that most of the child maltreatment cases involved the parents of the child, with more than half being the father of the child. From 1990 to 2004 the rate of child physical abuse and sexual abuse decreased, emotional abuse rates fluctuated, and the neglect rate increased, especially for children younger than 1 year. The study concluded that the trend for military families was similar to that of the general population.

One study found that the significant predictors of child abuse potential in Army mothers were depression, parental stress, family conflict, family cohesion, marital adjustment, and satisfaction with social support. For fathers the predictors were depression, parental stress, family conflict, and family expressiveness. One study investigated intimate partner violence in married women in the military, and found that women were more likely to be victims of violence from spouses.

Research on sexual stressors on functioning and psychiatric symptoms in active-duty men and women revealed that a greater percentage of women experienced sexual identity challenges, sexual harassment, and sexual assault. Those with more types of sexual stressors had more depression and anxiety, and more severe PTSD and somatic complaints. For former military reservist women from all branches of the service, sexual harassment was found to be associated with a greater risk of somatic symptoms, depression, and medical conditions. Studies have revealed that military sexual trauma was associated with PTSD, alcohol disorders, anxiety disorders, pain, obesity, starving behaviors, self-identifying as disabled, more severe symptoms and functional impairment, gynecologic symptoms, and suicide. Mediators of sexual assault were found in one study to be increased physical health-related quality of life, having a close partner, and lack of gynecologic morbidity.

"About one third of the population has a direct relationship with someone in the military."[26] Friends, families, and health care professionals need to be aware of the issues faced by military families. Health care for military families is not limited to the confines of the military health care system. Spouses and families of service members often receive care in the community where they live. Service members, spouses, and children attend schools and activities in the community. The interaction with service members and their families provides opportunities to recognize those who may be dealing with the effect of deployment, family violence, and military sexual trauma. Providing guidance and referral to appropriate health care providers is vital for the well-being of service members and military families.

A national initiative, *Joining Forces: Taking Action to Serve America's Military Families*,[27] was launched in April 2011by First Lady Michelle Obama and Dr Jill Biden. The purpose of *Joining Forces* is to mobilize society to support and provide opportunities for military service members and their families. A Web page on the *White House* web site details this new initiative and facilitates ways for Americans to become involved: http://www.whitehouse.gov/joiningforces.

Joining Forces identifies 3 areas of focus: employment, education, and wellness. Employment opportunities and military family–friendly workplaces for military spouses are one area of focus. Second, there is the need for educational institutions to be sensitive to the demands made on military families who need to move to new duty stations on a regular basis. Third, there should be a focus on wellness for service members and their families. The wellness aspect addresses the stress of war, deployments, and frequent moves of military families. It calls for the joining of forces to address the critical issues faced by military families and veterans, and to expand access to wellness programs and resources for service members and their families.

More research is needed to gain knowledge about the effect of deployment on military families, family violence, and military sexual trauma. Much of the current research is quantitative and retrospective. The use of a qualitative approach, such as descriptive phenomenology and prospective studies, both quantitative and qualitative, may reveal greater insight into how health care professionals can best provide care to military service members and their families.

REFERENCES

1. Sheppard SC, Malatras JW, Israel AC. The impact of deployment on U.S. military families. Am Psychol 2010;65:599–609.
2. Kimerling R, Street AE, Pavao J, et al. Military-related sexual trauma among Veterans Health Administration patients returning from Afghanistan. Am J Public Health 2010;100:1409–12.
3. Rentz ED, Martin SL, Gibbs DA, et al. Family violence in the military: a review of the literature. Trauma Violence Abuse 2006;7:93–108.
4. Palmer C. A theory of risk and resilience factors in military families. Mil Psychol 2008;20:205–17.
5. McCubbin HI, Patterson JM. The family stress process: the double ABCX model of adjustment and adaptation. Marriage Fam Rev 1983;6:7–37.
6. Patterson JM, McCubbin HI. The impact of family life events and changes on the health of a chronically ill child. Fam Relat 1983;32:255–64.
7. Bradley C. Veteran status and marital aggression: does military service make a difference? J Fam Violence 2007;22:197–209.
8. US Department of Veterans Affairs. VA Testimony of Bradley G. Mayes before Congress on May 20, 2010. Available at: http://www.va.gov/OCA/testimony/hvac/sdama/100520BGM.asp. Accessed April 15,2011.
9. Chapin M. Deployment and families: hero stories and horror stories. Smith Coll Stud Soc Work 2009;79:263–82.
10. Fonseca CA, Schmaling KB, Stoever C, et al. Variables associated with intimate partner violence in a deploying military sample. Mil Med 2006;171:627–31.
11. Warner CH, Appenzeller GN, Warner CM, et al. Psychological effects of deployments on military families. Psychiatr Ann 2009;39:56–63.
12. Barker LH, Berry KD. Developmental issues impacting military families with young children during single and multiple deployments. Mil Med 2009;174:1033–40.
13. Huebner AJ, Mancini JA, Wilcox RM, et al. Parental deployment and youth in military families: exploring uncertainty and ambiguous loss. Fam Relat 2007;56:112–22.
14. McCarroll JE, Fan Z, Newby JH, et al. Trends in US army child maltreatment reports: 1990-2004. Child Abuse Rev 2008;17:108–18.
15. Schaeffer CM, Alexander PC, Bethke K, et al. Predictors of child abuse potential among military parents: comparing mothers and fathers. J Fam Violence 2005;20:123–9.
16. Forgey MA, Badger L. Patterns of intimate partner violence among married women in the military: type, level, directionality and consequences. J Fam Violence 2006;21:369–80.
17. Suras A, Lind L. Military sexual trauma: a review of prevalence and associated health consequences in veterans. Trauma Violence Abuse 2008;9:250–69.

18. Murdoch M, Pryor JB, Polusny MA, et al. Functioning and psychiatric symptoms among military men and women exposed to sexual stressors. Mil Med 2007;172: 718–25.
19. Street AE, Stafford J, Mahan CM, et al. Sexual harassment and assault experienced by reservists during military service: prevalence and health correlates. J Rehabil Res Dev 2008;45:409–20.
20. Kimerling R, Gima K, Smith MW, et al. The Veterans Health Administration and military sexual trauma. Am J Public Health 2007;97:2160–6.
21. Haskell SG, Gordon KS, Mattocks K, et al. Gender differences in rates of depression, PTSD, pain, obesity, and military sexual trauma among Connecticut war veterans of Iraq and Afghanistan. J Womens Health (Larchmt) 2010;19:267–71.
22. Rowe EL, Gradus JL, Pineles SL, et al. Military sexual trauma in treatment-seeking women veterans. Mil Psychol 2009;21:387–95.
23. Campbell R, Lichty LF, Sturza M, et al. Gynecological health impact of sexual assault. Res Nurs Health 2006;29:399–413.
24. Belik SL, Stein MB, Asmundson GJ, et al. Relationship between traumatic events and suicide attempts in Canadian military personnel. Can J Psychiatry 2009;54: 93–104.
25. McCall-Hosenfeld JS, Liebschutz JM, Spiro A, et al. Sexual assault in the military and its impact on sexual satisfaction in women veterans: a proposed model. J Womens Health (Larchmt) 2009;18:901–9.
26. Park N. Military children and families: strengths and challenges during peace and war. Am Psychol 2011;66:65–72.
27. Joining Forces. Taking action to serve America's military families, 2011. Available at: http://www.whitehouse.gov/joiningforces. Accessed May 1, 2011.

Workplace Violence in Nursing Today

Susan Araujo, RN, MSN, NE-BC[a], Laura Sofield, RN, MSN, APN[b],*

KEYWORDS

- Verbal abuse
- Workplace violence
- Oppressed group behavior

WORKPLACE VIOLENCE IN NURSING TODAY: A FOCUS ON VERBAL ABUSE

Violence in nursing is not a new phenomenon. Various researchers (Refs.[1–3] and Araujo S, Sofield L. Verbal abuse of nurses and intent to leave. Unpublished dissertation, 2000, Kean University) in the last 2 decades have studied violence in nursing and have coined a definition of this condition. Studies have defined violence in slightly different ways, but the theme is similar. The World Health Organization (WHO)[4] defines violence as "the intentional use of physical force or power, threatened or actual, against oneself, another person or against a group or community that either results in or has a high likelihood of resulting in injury, death, psychological harm, maldevelopment or deprivation."

Serious perusal of this definition can uncover the many aspects of actual or potential violence for nurses today. The WHO begins the definition with "intentional use of physical force or power." Multiple studies (Araujo S, Sofield L. Verbal abuse of nurses and intent to leave. Unpublished dissertation, 2000, Kean University)[1,2,5] describe violence by many different perpetrators. Review of the perpetrators studied reveal patients to have been included in this class but the aspect of intention must be relevant to that individual. The studies[1,6] that define the patient as the perpetrator must address the mental state of the individual at the point of violence being perpetrated to be valid.

Threatened or actual violence is another important aspect of the WHO definition, which emphasizes that violence is not only the act of physical assault but emotional abuse as well. Although physical violence is heinous, verbal violence toward another is more ubiquitous. Verbal abuse occurs more frequently (Araujo S, Sofield L. Verbal abuse of nurses and intent to leave. Unpublished dissertation, 2000, Kean University) than physical violence and is more likely to be underreported. However, verbal assaults leave long-lasting impressions on the victim. The impressions left by this abuse can be similar to those found in posttraumatic stress disorder.[7]

The authors have nothing to disclose.
a Community Medical Center, 99 Route 37 West, Toms River, NJ 08755, USA
b Mid-Atlantic Geriatrics Association, 1205 Highway 35 North, Ocean, NJ 07712, USA
* Corresponding author.
E-mail address: Laura08723@comcast.net

Nurs Clin N Am 46 (2011) 457–464
doi:10.1016/j.cnur.2011.08.006
0029-6465/11/$ – see front matter © 2011 Elsevier Inc. All rights reserved.

The WHO further states that abuse may also be self-inflicted, and this may be the result of having been a victim of abuse leading to lowered self-esteem.

According to Collins,[8] "past victimization is a strong predictor of future abuse," so one abuser can produce many, and often lead to horizontal violence.

Horizontal violence in nursing is generally perpetrated by people with more perceived authority than their victims. An important aspect of this is the concept known as nurses eating their young, which is a phenomenon of this violence. Nurses eating their young is a symptom of oppressed group behavior, which is discussed later in this article. The WHO also addresses violence toward groups that is characterized by racial slurs, behavior toward nondominant groups, and those considered weaker or outside the mainstream or group norms.[9,10]

Violence may result in injury, death (physical violence), psychological harm, maldevelopment, or deprivation (verbal abuse). This article discusses all the aspects of violence in nursing, which include horizontal violence, vertical violence, and violence from patients, family, and visitors, as well verbal abuse.

According to the most recent statistics from the Bureau of Justice National Crime Victimization Survey[11] (NCVS), released in December 2001, between 1993 and 1999 an average of 1.7 million violent episodes per year were committed against workers. The profession most likely to be physically assaulted were police officers and the least likely to be physically assaulted were college professors. When comparing this with the medical profession, police officers experienced 260 violent victimizations per 1000 workers, college professors experienced 1.6 violent victimizations per 1000 workers, and nurses 21.9 episodes per 1000 workers. "The workplace violent crime victimization rate for nurses was not significantly different from that for physicians; however, nurses experienced workplace crime at a rate 72% higher than medical technicians and at more than twice the rate of other medical field workers."[11]

Within the medical profession, the highest incidence of victimization occurred in the mental health field, with professionals experiencing 68.2 episodes of violence per 1000 workers.

The time of day of victimization in heath care does not seem to be of any significance, with 52% of episodes occurring during the day and 44% occurring during the night.[11] According to the NCVS,[11] the health care worker is not likely to fight back during an assault but is more likely to use nonconfrontational tactics toward opponents. The survey also addresses violent crime but does not include those episodes in which physical violence was not a component. A more salient form of violence is verbal abuse, which often goes unreported but has lasting and psychologically damaging effects. Organizations such as The Joint Commission have mandated that all accredited health care organizations institute a new Leadership Standard that addresses disruptive and inappropriate behavior that may lead to medical errors, decreased patient satisfaction, increased cost of care, and reduced retention of nursing staff.[12]

Whitehorn and Nowland[13] in 1997, supported by Rippon[14] in 2000, reported that 65% to 82% of nursing staff have experienced verbal abuse. Although verbal abuse has been prevalent for many years, it has not received much attention. Research on verbal abuse in nursing (Araujo S, Sofield L. Verbal abuse of nurses and intent to leave. Unpublished dissertation, 2000, Kean University)[15,16] shows that many nurses historically have accepted such treatment and some have left the profession as a result of such victimization.

Verbal abuse leaves no visible scars; however, the emotional damage to the victim can be devastating.[17] Although there is no universal definition of verbal abuse, it can be overt or subtle.[18] It can encompass profanity, derogatory remarks, gossip, rumors, silence, sarcasm, labeling, blaming, and humorous put-downs.[17–19] Verbal abuse can be defined as a form of mistreatment, spoken or unspoken, that leaves its victim feeling personally or professionally attacked, devalued, or humiliated. It is communicated through words, tone, or a manner that disparages, intimidates, patronizes, threatens, accuses, or is disrespectful toward another (Araujo S, Sofield L. Verbal abuse of nurses and intent to leave. Unpublished dissertation, 2000, Kean University).[20,21]

Some of the causes of verbal abuse in the health care setting are related to the stressful situations and the power differentials present. Verbal abuse occurs between nurses and their patients, families, physicians, immediate supervisors, and peers.[15,22,23] According to Diaz and McMillin,[22] it is an inappropriate use of power by someone in a dominant position toward an actual or perceived subordinate through words, tone, manner, or other nonverbal means. Vertical violence is best shown by the nurse-physician relationship. Nurses have long been yielding power to physicians by being acquiescent in their communication.

Power creates a gulf between physicians and nurses. Although they work closely together and share common goals, nurses have always taken a subservient role.[24] This perception by nurses that the physician is omnipotent has created unequal interpersonal relationships.[25] Nurses have always believed themselves to be powerless, with the physician being the only powerful player in the health care arena. However, nurses have enormous power to influence the welfare of their patients.[18] Conversely, according to Roche and colleagues,[26] an unsafe working environment can have damaging effects on patient outcomes. The inappropriate use of power by the physician creates an atmosphere of stress in the professional relationship.[23]

Stress increases the prevalence of verbal abuse. For patients and families, stress is caused by the lack of control experienced. This stress is exacerbated by the dwindling resources available to nursing staff, which in turn causes a delay in meeting patient needs, causing more frustration for both the patient and nurse. As stress increases, verbal abuse escalates, leading to an increased potential for job dissatisfaction and increasing the likelihood that nurses will leave the profession. A vicious cycle is created as staff turnover leads to more stressful environments. Nurses have accepted verbal abuse from patients and their families as part of the job, and reporting it has not been considered worthwhile for fear of being reprimanded or accused of not providing appropriate care.[10,27]

Patients' opinions of care have been a target of increasing scrutiny. Center for Medicare and Medicaid Services (CMS) 2010[28] has developed the Hospital Consumer Assessment of Healthcare Providers and Systems (HCAHPS) Survey. HCAHPS is a survey to measure patients' perceptions of their hospital experience, and is a public report. Beginning in 2013, 30% of hospital Medicare reimbursement will be tied to HCAHPS results, which has placed additional stress on the nursing staff in hospitals to meet the service needs of patients. HCAHPS surveys will be introduced in other health care settings, including outpatient and long-term care venues, in the next several years.

A 1982 study by Duldt[23] showed that nurses have a 50-50 chance of encountering verbal abuse during a week at work. In a landmark 1985 study, Cox[1] found that 77% of nurse managers and 82% of staff nurses have encountered abusive communication. The percentage of nurses affected by verbal abuse had increased to 97% of nurse managers and 96.7% of staff nurses when Cox[29] repeated her study in 1989. These findings were validated by Manderino and Berkey's[30] study, in which 90% of staff nurses surveyed reported an average of 6 to 12 episodes of verbal abuse in 1 year. Similar results were reported in studies by Zigrossi,[21] Diaz and McMillin,[22] Braun and colleagues,[15] and Araujo and Sofield (Araujo S, Sofield L. Verbal abuse of nurses and intent to leave. Unpublished dissertation, 2000, Kean University).

Studies have shown that verbal abuse significantly affects the workplace by decreasing morale, increasing job dissatisfaction, and creating a hostile work environment.[1,30] Cox[1] showed that at least 16% of nursing turnover is directly related to these factors. Bush and Gillilland[31] and Danesh and colleagues[6] contend that verbal abuse negates a caring organizational culture and threatens the organization itself by higher turnover rates, increased number of lawsuits, unionization, decreased productivity, increased errors, and overall decreased quality of care.

Verbal abuse has been noted to be a factor in nurses' intent to leave the organization and possibly the profession. Failure of the organization, and the profession itself, to provide the necessary support increases the already impending nursing crisis. Although there are studies on verbal abuse, they are limited. It has been suggested by researchers (Araujo S, Sofield L. Verbal abuse of nurses and intent to leave. Unpublished dissertation, 2000, Kean University)[29,32,33] that verbal abuse studies should be continued to better understand the correlation between verbal abuse and intent to leave the organization.

Nursing, with the assistance of the organization, must learn to create an environment that reinforces the value and retention of nurses. Failure to address the issue of verbal abuse places an organization at risk to increased turnover and cost resulting from decreased productivity and job satisfaction.[1,20,23,31] Although turnover cannot be totally avoided, when the cause of the turnover stems from problems within the organization, this creates a priority concern. Nursing turnover is costly to the organization. Jones and Gates[34] reported that the cost of replacing a nurse was as high as $64,000. The cost of turnover cannot simply be measured by the salary of the lost employee because other factors are also involved. Some of the factors included in the overall cost of nursing turnover include recruitment, orientation, agency usage, decreased productivity, increased patient errors, and a dysfunctional organizational culture.[34,35]

In addition to the fiscal implications of turnover, the impact on productivity becomes even more costly. Disruption of team functioning, introduction of new staff not knowledgeable about the ways of the organization, and changing interpersonal dynamics on the work team have all been shown to negatively affect work performance and work satisfaction. This effect becomes magnified in the summative effect of turnover along with the presence of a work environment in which nurses believe themselves to be devalued and generally not supported. Research has positively correlated work satisfaction with patient satisfaction, so there is a deleterious snowball effect of a negative work environment on turnover in the institution.

Despite this awareness, more money continues to be spent on nurse recruitment rather than nurse retention.[36] As health care reenters a period in which critical shortages in nursing personnel are occurring or anticipated, the futility of emphasizing recruitment rather than retention becomes apparent. The prudent approach is to examine strategies to increase retention of staff. Because verbal abuse is a documented factor in turnover, and because verbal abuse has been linked to decreased productivity and decreased nurse satisfaction, which has been linked to decreased patient satisfaction, the issue of verbal abuse in the workplace must be further explored.

In addition to the general issues of support, administrators need to be more attentive to the potential liability that can result from verbal abuse. Employees may take legal action against the organization for comments related to gender, religion, ethnic background, or age, because these remarks can be considered discriminatory.[6] The health care system suffers along with its employees from the cost of correcting errors, offsetting absenteeism, resignations, and compromised care. Calculating the cost of defending 1 lawsuit or of contending with a union in a complaint that relates to verbal abuse could show the economic damage done by verbal abuse.[29] Not only is the damage monetary, but the effect on the patient/nurse/physician relationship can be severe.

When verbal abuse is witnessed by the patient or family, the reaction of patients and families to this unprofessional behavior can be to question the ability of the health care team to safely and competently render quality care.[29] Diaz and McMillin[22] state that these types of interactions decrease the credibility of the nurse and the respect for the physician, increase the sense of helplessness in the patient, and severely alter the quality of consumer opinion for these 2 health care delivery groups. Sheridan-Leos[37] found that patients and families make more complaints in organizations in which verbal abuse is prevalent. Other negative factors besides compromised care are decreased productivity, morale, and job satisfaction, as well as increased turnover and the possibility of unionization. On an individual basis, the cost to the nurse is great because it diminishes self-esteem, leads to a lack of collaboration and teamwork, and promotes negative attitudes, depression, and confidence.[38] The effects on the nurse lead to conduct that is consistent with oppressed group behavior.

The nursing profession has developed its own culture. However, much of that culture shows a propensity toward oppressed group behavior. Not only does the nursing profession exhibit the characteristics of this group, it shows a lack of cohesion and support for peers and the profession in general. This behavior creates a vicious cycle, perpetuating the oppressed group behavior model. Oppressed group behavior has been defined by Roberts[39] as being shown by persons who are in groups that are subordinate to more powerful groups in their society learning certain behavior patterns that, although necessary for survival, lead to a cycle of further oppression. Marginality, which is part of the oppressed group behavior, causes nurses to take on the characteristics of the oppressor while losing their individual identities, which leads to frustration and negative self-image.[40] Nursing's negative self-opinion stems from being defined as inferior by other members of the health care team, and verbally abusive encounters strengthen this perception.

Studies of oppressed groups date back to literature on colonized Africans and Latin Americans, the American Negro, Jews, and, more recently, women.[41–43] Paulo Freire[44] describes the major characteristics of oppressed groups developing as a result of a dominant group's ability to have their norms and values seen as the right ones. The dominant group norms are internalized by the subordinate group, who believe that, by being like the dominant group, they hold the same power and status.

Those who are successful at internalizing the dominant group's behavior and norms are considered to be marginalized. These group members do not fit into the dominant group and can not be considered members of the subordinate group; they instead lose their own identity. The loss of identity often leads to low self-esteem and to self-hatred, which perpetuates the oppression by the dominant group.

This continued oppression creates feelings that lead to what has been termed submissive-aggression syndrome.[45] The subordinate group becomes submissive to the dominant group but aggressive to members of its own culture, leading to horizontal violence or anger directed toward self and peers.

Nursing can be viewed as an oppressed group because they have internalized the values of the physician and the medical model. Nursing, and especially nursing leadership, has been encouraged to look like a physician and look to medicine for support. This kind of leadership leads to competition among nurses and a lack of cohesion in the profession. The growth of such terms as nurses eating their young result from this oppressed behavior.[46] It has been well documented that nurses underreport verbal abuse.[9,16,47–49] This underreporting stems from oppressed behavior because nurses blame themselves for the abuse instead of placing the blame on the abuser, which leads to nurses accepting verbal abuse from all sources as part of the job. They do not think that they have the power to prevent such events.

Verbal abuse then becomes a coping mechanism as nurses directs their frustration inwardly, toward each other, themselves, and perceived subordinates.[50,51] This horizontal violence is related to the nurse's lack of autonomy, accountability, and control of the nursing profession.[49] Applying research based on the framework of oppressed group behavior by Roberts[49] to the area of verbal abuse will therefore allow a health care system to better understand where education needs to be focused. Through education and policy implementation, an organization can effectively empower its nurses to eliminate verbal abuse.

Although there have been zero-tolerance policies, education related to violence in the workplace, and a more open dialogue related to verbal abuse in health care organizations, little has been accomplished to stop this phenomenon. As discussed in this article, many studies have addressed verbal abuse in the past 2 decades and several have suggested strategies for prevention; however, more work is needed.

If administrators are going to create supportive environments with zero tolerance for verbal abuse, then the behavioral manifestations of verbal abuse in the health care system must be better understood. By studying this phenomenon, it is possible to identify the prevalence and sources of verbal abuse within a system and develop programs to assist nurses to deal with the feelings it creates and to develop system strategies for an environment with zero tolerance for verbal abuse.

REFERENCES

1. Cox HC. Verbal abuse in nursing: report of a study. Nurs Manag 1987;18(11): 47–50.
2. Anderson C. Workplace violence: are some nurses more vulnerable? Issues Ment Health Nurs 2002;23:351–66.
3. Howard PK, Gilboy N. Workplace violence. Adv Emerg Nurs J 2009;31(2): 94–100.
4. Krug EG, Dahlberg LL, Mercy JA, et al, editors. World report on violence and health. Geneva (Switzerland): World Health Organization; 2002.
5. Farrell GA. Aggression in clinical settings; nurses' views – a follow up study. J Adv Nurs 1999;29(3):532–41.
6. Danesh VC, Mulvey D, Fottler MD. Hidden workplace violence; what your nurses may not be telling you. Health Care Manag 2008;27(4):357–63.
7. Brennan W. Sounding off about verbal abuse. Occupational Health 2003;55(11): 22–7.
8. Collin M. Factors influencing sexual victimization and revictimization in a sample of adolescent mothers. J Interpers Violence 1998;13(2):3–25.
9. Martin A, Gray C, Adam A. Nurses' responses to workplace verbal abuse, a scenario study of the impact of situational and individual factor. Res Pract Hum Resource Manag 2007;1–22.
10. Gates DM, Kroeger D. Violence against nurses: the silent epidemic. ISNA Bulletin 2002-2003;29(1):1–21.
11. Bureau of Justice Statistics Special Report National Crime Victimization Survey; violence in the workplace, 1993-1999. 2001. NCJ, 190076. Available at: http://www.ojp.usdoj.gov/bjsl/. Accessed August 3, 2011.

12. The Joint Commission. Sentinel event alert; behaviors that undermine a culture of safety. Available at: http://www.jointcommission.org/sentineleventsalert/sentinal eventalert/sea_40.htm. Accessed on February 28, 2011.
13. Whitehorn D, Nowland M. Towards an aggression-free healthcare environment. Can Nurse 1997;93:24–6.
14. Rippon TJ. Aggression and violence in healthcare professional. J Adv Nurs 2000; 31:452–60.
15. Braun K, Christel D, Walker D, et al. Verbal abuse of nurses and nonnurses. Nurs Manag 1991;22(3):72–6.
16. Lybecker C. Violence against nurses: a silent epidemic. Workplace Violence Prevention Reporter. Vancouver, BC (Canada): Specialty Technical Publishers (STP); 1998. p. 1–3.
17. Elgin SH. The gentle art of self defense. Englewood Cliffs (NJ): Prentice Hall; 1980.
18. Cooper A, Saxe-Braithwite M, Anthony R. Verbal abuse of hospital staff. Can Nurse 1996;92(6):31–4.
19. Whittington R, Shuttleworth S, Hill L. Violence to staff in a general hospital setting. J Adv Nurs 1996;24:326–33.
20. Nield-Anderson L, Clarke JT. De-escalating verbal aggression in primary care settings. Nurse Pract 1996;21(10):95–107.
21. Zigrossi ST. Verbal behaviors perceived as abusive by hospital staff nurses and supervisors and influence on intent to leave the organization [dissertation]. Rochester (NY): University of Rochester; 1992. p. 1–121.
22. Diaz A, McMillan JD. A definition and description of nurse abuse. West J Nurs Res 1991;13(1):97–109.
23. Duldt BW. Anger: an alienating communication hazard for nurses. Nurs Outlook 1982;640–4.
24. Schmalenberg C, Kramer M. Nurse-physician relationships in hospitals: 20000 nurses tell their story. Crit Care Nurse 2009;29(1):74–83.
25. Rosenstein AH, Russell H, Lauve R. Disruptive physician behavior contributes to nursing shortage: study links bad behavior by doctors to nurse's leaving the profession. Physician Exec 2002;28(6):8–11.
26. Roche M, Diers D, Duffield C, et al. Violence towards nurses, the work environment and patient outcomes. J Nurs Scholarsh 2010;42(1):13–22.
27. Ferns T, Chojnacka I. Reporting incidence of violence and aggression towards NHS staff. Nurs Stand 2005;19:51–6.
28. Center for Medicare & Medicaid Services. What is CAHPS? Available at: http://www.cms.gov Accessed on February 28, 2011.
29. Cox HC. Verbal abuse nationwide part 2: impact and modification. Nurs Manag 1991;20(3):66–9.
30. Manderino MA, Berkey N. Verbal abuse of staff nurses by physicians. J Prof Nurs 1997;13(1):48–55.
31. Bush HA, Gilliland M. Enhancing a quality culture by managing verbal abuse. Nurs Qual Connect 1995;4(4):5.
32. Cox HC. Verbal abuse nationwide part 1: oppressed group behavior. Nurs Manag 1991;22(2):32–5.
33. Hilton PE, Kottke J, Pfabler D. Verbal abuse in nursing: how serious is it? Nurs Manag 1992;25(5):90.
34. Jones CB, Gates M. The cost and benefits of nurse turnover: a business case for nurse retention. Online J Issues Nurs 2007;12(3). Manuscript 4.
35. Obrien-Pallas LL, Thomson D, McGillis Hall L, et al. Evidence-based standards for measuring staff nursing and performance. Available at: http://www.hhrchair.ca/images/CMSImages?EBS%20full%20report.pdf. Accessed February 28, 2011.

36. Jolma DJ. Relationships between nursing workload and turnover. Nurs Econ 1990;8(2):110–4.
37. Sheridan-Leos N. Understanding lateral violence in nursing. Clin J Oncol Nurs 2008;12(13):399–403.
38. Patterson P. Disruptive behavior. OR Manager 1996;12(12):8–9.
39. Roberts SJ. Point of view: breaking the cycle of oppression: lessons for nurse practitioners. J Am Acad Nurse Pract 1996;8(5):209–14.
40. St-Pierre I, Holmes D. Managing nurses through disciplinary power: a Foucauldian analysis of workplace violence. J Nurs Manag 2008;16:352–9.
41. Carmichael S, Hamilton C. Black power. New York: Random House; 1967.
42. Ehrenreich B, English D. For her own good. Garden City (NY): Anchor Press; 1979.
43. Memmi A. The colonizer and the colonized. New York (NY): Orion Press; 1995.
44. Freire P. Pedagogy of the oppressed. New York: Heider and Heider; 1971.
45. Fanon F. The wretched of the Earth. New York: Gove Press; 1963.
46. Rowe MM, Sherlock H. Stress and verbal abuse in nursing: do burned out nurses eat their young? J Nurs Manag 2005;13:242–8.
47. American Nurses Association (ANA). Workplace violence: can you close the door on it? American Nurses Association; 1994. Available at: http://www.nursingworld.org/dlwa/osh/wp5.htm. p. 1–4. Accessed February 28, 2011.
48. Elliott P. Violence in health care: what nurse managers need to know. Nurs Manag 1997;1–7. Available at: http://www.springnet.com/ce/m712a.htm#health. Accessed February 28, 2011.
49. Roberts SJ. Oppressed group behavior: implications for nursing. Adv Nurs Sci 1983;5(4):21–30.
50. Cox HC. Excising verbal abuse. Today's OR Nurse 1994;16(1):38–40.
51. McCall E. Horizontal violence in nursing: the continuing silence. Lamp 1996; 53(3):28–9.

The Impact of Interpersonal Violence on Health Care

Rose Knapp, DNP, RN, APN-C

KEYWORDS

- Interpersonal violence • Intimate partner violence • Child abuse
- Elder abuse

Violence kills millions of people each year. The impact of interpersonal violence is pervasive in today's society and results in long-term physical, psychological, economic, and social consequences. The World Health Organization (WHO)[1] and Centers for Disease Control (CDC)[2] identify acts of interpersonal violence as family or community violence. Family violence is categorized by the victim: child, intimate partner, or elder.[3] Child abuse is defined by the WHO[1] and CDC[2] as physical, sexual, and emotional abuse, and neglect. Intimate partner violence (IPV) occurs between two partners involved in a close relationship. Intimate partners are defined by the CDC[4] as current or former spouses or dating partners. Elder abuse is defined as mistreatment of older people over the age of 60 years in the home or institutional setting.[3]

The medical and economic impact of interpersonal violence is overwhelming. The US Department of Health and Human Services Administration for Children and Families[5] reported that, in 2008, 772,000 children in the United States were maltreated with more than 3.7 million investigations or assessments conducted. IPV has resulted in 4.8 million physical assaults and rapes of women and of 2.9 million men. The medical, mental health care, and lost productivity costs, according to the CDC,[4] rose from 5.8 billion in 1995 to 8.3 billion in 2003. It is believed that these numbers are much higher because many victims of IPV do not report the violence because of their fear of the abuser and the feeling that no one can help them out of their unfortunate situation. The economic impact of IPV is attributed to unemployment, increased job turnover, increased need for disability and welfare, and decreased income of the victims.

According to the United Nations Elder Population Division,[6] there will be an estimated 1.2 billion individuals over the age of 60 by the year 2025. It must be a priority to establish strategies to protect this vulnerable population. The National Center for Victims of Crimes[7] reports that, in 2004, Adult Protective Services received 565,747

Marjorie K. Unterberg School of Nursing and Health Studies, Monmouth University, 400 Cedar Avenue, West Long Branch, NJ 07764, USA
E-mail address: rknapp@monmouth.edu

Nurs Clin N Am 46 (2011) 465–470
doi:10.1016/j.cnur.2011.08.004
0029-6465/11/$ – see front matter © 2011 Elsevier Inc. All rights reserved.

reports of elder abuse and that 191,908 of these reports were substantiated. The economic impact of resultant emergency department visits, hospitalizations, and required treatments (eg, medications, physical therapy), and required follow-up of elder abuse must be researched and prevention strategies must be implemented. All three types of interpersonal abuse are on the rise and it is import for health care providers to increase their awareness and for institutes to put into place initiatives to decrease the incidence of violent mistreatments of these vulnerable populations.

CHILD MALTREATMENT

Child maltreatment as defined by the CDC[8] includes all types of abuse of a child under the age of 18 by a parent, caregiver, or another person of custodial care such as a member of the clergy, coach, or teacher. The four types of abuse include (1) physical abuse or the use of force, such as hitting, kicking, shaking, burning, or other show of force; (2) sexual abuse and engaging in sexual acts, including fondling or exposing a child to sexual acts; (3) emotional abuse, including harm to the child's self-worth or emotional well-being, such as name-calling, shaming, rejection, withholding love, and threatening; and (4) neglect, failure to meet the child's basic needs, including housing, food, clothing, education, and access to health care.

The US Department of Health and Human Services Administration for Children and Families[1] reports that, in 2008, 38.3% of perpetrators of child fatalities were the child's mother; 18.9%, fathers; and 17.9%, both parents. Parents, therefore, accounted for 75.1% of the violent deaths of children. Of these fatalities, 39.7% were caused by multiple forms of maltreatment; 31.9%, neglect; 22.9%, physical abuse; 1.5%, medical neglect; 1.3%, psychological neglect; 0.4%, sexual abuse; and 2.3%, other. The victims were more prevalent among children in lower socioeconomic families. The incidence of African American child fatality was twice that of white non-Hispanic children.[1] The CDC[8] identifies those factors that predispose a child to mistreatment. Children under the age of 4 years are at a greater risk for severe injury and death. Another contributing factor is environments in which the family is under a great deal of stress from drug or alcohol abuse, poverty, and/or chronic health problems. The community environment that does not reject child abuse significantly contributes to the perpetuation of child maltreatment.

Severe injuries in children under the age of 4 years can take many forms and require astute assessment by health care providers. Usually serious damage is the result of head injury or injury to the internal organs.[5] Head injury is the most common cause of death. Suspicion of abuse is further warranted when fractures occur in bones that are rarely broken under normal circumstances, such as a femur in an infant who is yet to walk. Shaking an infant is another prevalent form of abuse in young children. Approximately one-third of severely shaken infants die and most survivors suffer mental retardation, cerebral palsy, or blindness. According to the WHO, a battered child presenting repeatedly with inflicted, devastating injuries is a tragic but fortunately statistically a rare occurrence.[5]

Recognizing sexual abuse requires a high index of suspicion and familiarity of the subtle, indirect physical and behavioral indicators of abuse. Children who are sexually abused rarely exhibit the obvious signs of abuse such as signs of genitourinary infection, genital injury, abdominal pain, or overt behavioral problems. The signs of abuse are more subtle. Neglect may manifest as noncompliance, failure to seek medical treatment, deprivation of food, poor hygiene, and the failure of a child to physically thrive. Exposure to environmental dangers is also a form of neglect, including exposure to drugs, unsafe living conditions, and inadequate adult supervision. Neglect also includes abandonment and being deprived of an education.

IPV

IPV has a profound impact on health care. As previously stated, it accounts for 8.3 billion dollars in health care expenditures. IPV occurs between two persons in a close relationship. CDC[4] defines an intimate partner as a current or former spouse or dating partner. The WHO[1] identifies four types of IPV behavior. These include (1) physical violence in which a person hurts or tries to hurt a partner by hitting, kicking, or any type of physical force; (2) sexual violence, such as forcing a partner to take part in a sex act without their permission; (3) physical or sexual threats, in which words, gestures, weapons, or other means are used to communicate a threat; and (4) emotional abuse, such as threats toward a partner or their possessions or loved ones, or harm of a person's sense of self-worth by stalking, name-calling, or preventing a partner to see loved ones. Frequently, IPV starts with emotional abuse and then escalates to physical or sexual abuse, or these may occur simultaneously.[4]

IPV has a significant impact on the victim's health. Physical ailments, such as abdominal and thoracic injuries, abrasions, lacerations, chronic pain, fibromyalgia, fractures, gastrointestinal disorders, irritable bowel disorders, and ocular damage may occur because of IPV. Sexual and reproductive disorders are also prevalent among victims of IPV and include infertility, pelvic inflammatory disease, pregnancy complications and/or miscarriage, sexual dysfunction, sexually transmitted diseases, and unwanted pregnancy. Psychologically, IPV may lead to alcohol and substance abuse, depression and anxiety, eating and sleeping disorders, poor self-esteem, posttraumatic stress disorder, smoking, unsafe sexual behavior, and suicidal behavior.[1,4] Humphries and Lee[9] studied 346 ethnically diverse women living in California to identify IPV exposure. A history of physical or sexual abuse was reported by 33% of the women and at least 20% reported both types of abuse. The women, regardless of their ethnicity and socioeconomic status, reported an increase in IPV-associated chronic health problems and depression. The women also cited difficulty in expressing their concerns about their abuse with friends or family because of fear of being labeled as a victim of abuse. Some women who stayed in the abusive relationship also reported the fear of leaving the financial support (ie, loss of income) if they left.

The WHO and CDC identify the demographics of the perpetrators of abuse, including a young age, heavy alcohol drinking, substance abuse, depression, low academic achievement, and witnessing violence or being a victim of violence during childhood.[1,4] The perpetrator of abuse may be experiencing a life event that is causing increased stress, such as unemployment or financial difficulties. The perpetrator of IPV may be undergoing a relationship or marital conflict, such as economic stress.[9] Krug and colleagues[10] further identify the risk factors for becoming a victim or perpetrator of violence.

Individual Factors

1. Victim of child abuse and neglect
2. Psychological or personality disorder
3. Physical health disabilities
4. Abuse of alcohol or other substances, or gun ownership.

Relationship factors

1. Marital conflicts around gender roles
2. Association with friends who engage in violent behavior
3. Poor parenting practices

4. Parental conflict involving the use of violence
5. Low socioeconomic status.

Community factors
1. High residential mobility
2. High unemployment
3. Social isolation
4. Proximity to drug trade
5. Poverty
6. Weak community support system.

ELDER MALTREATMENT

Increased life expectancy, attributable to advances in medical technology, has contributed to the increased number of older adults in the United States. Elder abuse and maltreatment have become more prevalent. In 2004, Adult Protective Services reported a 16% increase from their previous 2000 survey of all 50 states.[7] Previously, in other generations, older adults were cared for by their extended family who shared in the responsibilities. Elder abuse may be attributed to societal changes, such as strained economic times, smaller nuclear families, and increased mobility of family members.

Elder abuse is divided into five categories.[7,11] First, physical abuse includes nonaccidental physical force that results an injury. Indicators include fractures and dislocations, lacerations, abrasions, burns, head injuries, and bruises to upper arms, wrist and ankles, or thighs. Second, sexual abuse indicators include sexually transmitted disease and pain, itching, bleeding, or bruising in the genital area. Third, psychological abuse indicators include low self-esteem, being overly anxious or withdrawn, extreme changes in mood, depression, or suicidal behavior. Fourth, neglect indicators include poor personal hygiene, signs of overmedication, medication misuse, being dressed in soiled clothing, being left alone and deprived of sensory stimulation, and malnutrition. Negligence can include active (willful) or passive failure to provide care, or self-neglect (failure of elder to care for themselves).[7,11] Fifth, financial abuse includes theft or exploitation of money or property accomplished by force or illegal means, including illegally misusing an elder's money or assets. This form of abuse may manifest as cashing of checks without authorization or permission, forging a signature, or improper use of power of attorney or guardianship. Frequently, the abuser is the person who is directly responsible for the care of the older adult and someone who they depend on or care for deeply.[11] The maltreatment of elder population directly affects the physical and psychological health of this vulnerable population. The increasing number of abused elders directly affects health care costs, so strategies to prevent potentially abusive situations must be a public health priority initiative.

STRATEGIES TO PREVENT INTERPERSONAL VIOLENCE
Preventing Child Maltreatment

The ultimate goal of preventing child maltreatment is to institute strategies that support parents, programs to provide family social support, and positive parenting. Positive parenting skills include responding to a child's needs, good communication, and appropriate discipline.[8] Rosenberg and colleagues[3] cited the importance of the following to help decrease child maltreatment: reduction of unintended pregnancies, prenatal care, treatment programs for children of violence, preschool enrichment programs, school-based programs to prevent child mistreatment, gun safety programs, home visitation services, mentoring, quality after school programs, recreational programs, and improved screening by health care providers.

Preventing IPV

The goal of ending IPV is attained by preventing it before it begins. A preventative approach is to implement programs that teach young people dating and healthy relationship skills. Because IPV is so closely tied to socioeconomic stressors, Rosenberg and colleagues[3] identified the following strategies to prevent the stressors that contribute to IPV: individual counseling, academic achievement programs, peer-mediation, family therapy, recreational programs, incentives for postsecondary school or vocational training, services for adults who were abused as children, and couples therapy.

Preventing Elder Abuse

The CDC[11] suggests strategies to prevent elder abuse, including listening to elders and their caregivers, reporting suspected abuse to Adult Protective Services, differentiating elder abuse from the normal aging process, involving a trusted professional in managing financial matters, finding an adult day care program, and using support systems and counseling. Fulmer and Greenberg[12] promote an interdisciplinary assessment and intervention plan as vital to ensure a safe environment for the older adult. Strategies they recommend include implementing a safety plan (eg, safe home placement), providing the elder with emergency telephone numbers and referrals, maximizing the elder's ability to communicate (ie, assuring access to eyeglasses and hearing aids), and regularly accessing the elder's caregiver for stress. To prevent financial abuse, they suggest utilizing direct deposit to avoid the handling of the elders money by others. They also stress the importance of developing a strategic plan with a set timeline to evaluate the management of the elder's finances and personal effects. Starr[6] stresses the importance of elder abuse education for those caring for the elderly population as a critical element to prevention. The education program should be focused on the forensic, financial, and legal aspects of abuse. This program would empower all persons involved in the care of elders to identify and report elder abuse.

SUMMARY

Interpersonal violence is prevalent in our society. Unfortunately, given the current stressors on individuals, families, and communities, the incidences of child abuse, IPV, and elder abuse are increasing. The economic impact on health care costs is significant. There are many contributing factors to abuse and they are all public health issues that must be addressed for these abuses to cease. The literature indicates that the profile of a perpetrator of abuse is a person who might have witnessed or been a victim of abuse as a child; has a limited education; has personality or psychological disorders; has personal stressors, such as limited income, unemployment, family, or marital discord; or has low self-esteem.

The health care provider must have the assessment skills to recognize the victims of child abuse, IPV, and elder abuse. Nurses must take a leadership role to assure that interpersonal violence and the strategies for prevention become a requirement in the curriculum of nursing schools. As leaders in health care, nurses should take a leadership role to implement antiviolence teaching and prevention programs in the community and patient population. Nurse leaders must also be aware of how cultural beliefs relate to interpersonal violence. By acknowledging cultural values and their differences, nurses will be able to successfully implement culturally appropriate strategies.[13]

As a society, it is our obligation to institute strategies to protect the victims of abuse, including funding women's and family shelters, providing after school programs in at-risk neighborhoods, and providing counseling to victims of abuse. We need to continue our commitment to convicting perpetrators of child abuse, IPV, and elder abuse. Programs must also be instituted to counsel and rehabilitate perpetrators of abuse. Community and religious programs should include emphasis on enabling families to deal with the problem of partner violence. Other community or school-based programs should include tackling youth violence, teenage pregnancies, substance abuse, and family violence.

It is the duty of society to promote optimal health and well-being of all citizens. The pervasive increase in numbers of the victims of interpersonal abuse resulting in exorbitant health care costs and fatalities necessitates concerted initiative and funding by both our government agencies and health care providers to eradicate abuse of vulnerable citizens.

REFERENCES

1. Waters H, Hyder A, Rajkotia Y, et al. The economic dimensions of interpersonal violence. Geneva (Switzerland): Department of Injuries and Violence Prevention, World Health Organization; 2004.
2. The Centers for Disease Control. Violence Prevention. Available at: http://www.cdc.gov/ViolencePrevention/globalviolence/. Accessed April 14, 2011.
3. Rosenberg M, Butchart A, Marcy J, et al. Interpersonal Violence in Disease Prevention Priorities in Developing Countries. Washington, DC: Oxford University Press; 2006. p. 755–69. Chapter 40.
4. The Centers for Disease Control. Understanding Intimate Partner Violence. Available at: http://www.cdc.gov/violenceprevention/ipv/. Accessed March 20, 2011.
5. Department of Health and Human Services, Administration on Children, Youth and Families. Child Maltreatment 2008. 2010. Available at: http://www.acf.hhs.gov. Accessed March 20, 2011.
6. Starr L. Preparing those caring for older adults to report elder abuse. J Contin Educ Nurs 2010;41(5):231–5.
7. National Center on Elder Abuse, 2004 Survey of State Adult Protective Services. Abuse of adult 60 years of age and older, prepared for the National Council on Elder Abuse, Oxford University Press, Washington, DC; 2006. vol. 2(2).
8. The Centers for Disease Control. Understanding child mistreatment. Available at: http://www.cdc.gov/violenceprevention/childmaltreatment/. Accessed March 20, 2011.
9. Humphries J, Lee K. Interpersonal violence is associated with depression and chronic physical health problem in midlife women. Issues Ment Health Nurs 2009;30:206–13.
10. Krug EG, Dahlberg I, Mercy Zwi AB, et al. World report on violence and health. Geneva: World Health Organization; 2002. p. 243–60.
11. The Centers for Disease Control. Understanding elder maltreatment. Available at: http://www.cdc.gov/violenceprevention/eldermaltreatment/. Accessed March 20, 2011.
12. Fulmer T, Greenberg S, Elder mistreatment and abuse. The Hartford Institute of Geriatric Nursing. Available at: http://consultgerirn.org/topics/elder_mistreatment_and_abuse/want_to_know_more. Accessed March 16, 2011.
13. Zoucha R. Considering culture in understanding interpersonal violence. J Forensic Nurs 2006;2(4):195–6.

The U.S. Department of Health & Human Services Administration for Children & Families has a toll-free crisis hotline, "Childhelp" (800-422-4453) hotline is a nonprofit organization that was originally funded by Sara O'Meara and Yvonne Fedderson it has a 24 hour hotline for children to call who are being abused physically. For child sexual abuse, they have a hotline called "Darkness to Light" (513) 460-4658 is a nonprofit service founded by Anne Lee is also a nonprofit organization its headquarters are in South Carolina and they train adults to prevent, recognize and react to childhood sexual abuse.[7] Most states have a child protection or child welfare agency within their Department of Children and Families. These agencies are responsible for investigating allegations of child abuse and neglect. They also arrange for the child's protection and the family's treatment if necessary. These agencies are often connected with community-based agencies throughout to provide services to children and families. These services may include counseling, parenting skills classes, substance abuse treatment, in-home services, foster care, and residential services. Often these agencies must work with the family court system.[8] Each state keeps data on their number of cases of maltreatment reported.[8]

Intimate Partners

The terms *intimate partner violence* (IPV) and *intimate partner abuse* (IPA) can be used interchangeably. Other terms used are *domestic violence* or *spouse abuse*. In a study published in 2010, researchers found that police filed 1607 incidents of IPV against women younger than 23 years. One-tenth of these women were younger than 18 years. Although their risk of police-documented IPV was lower, adolescents' experiences of IPV were remarkably similar to those of 18- to 22-year-olds'. As with adult victims, most assaults against adolescents were through bodily force (94.4%) and occurred in a private residence (75%). A substantial percentage of adolescent minorities were in adult-like relationships; 9% were married, 13.3% were cohabiting, and 20.25% had a child in common. A higher proportion of adolescents, however, experienced an aggravated (vs simple) assault (11.1%) and sustained visible injuries (12.1%).[9]

In 2008, another study looked at intimate violence among women in midlife and older women. The National Crime Victimization Survey showed that although the highest rates of nonlethal violence, including sexual and physical assault, were committed against younger women, the smaller percentage of victimized women were older than 55 years (2%). These findings translate to approximately 118,000 female victims between the years 1993 and 2000.[10] Women in this group of 620 reported being on public assistance and had a recent history of homelessness. In addition, these victims reported higher frequencies of HIV risk factors than nonvictims, including having a partner who insisted on sex without a condom, having sex with a man they knew or suspected was an intravenous drug user, and experiencing symptoms of or being diagnosed with or treated for a sexually transmitted infection. Significantly higher percentages of abused women reported being tested for HIV and being HIV seropositive. The National Violence Against Women survey showed that 0.2% of female respondents reported being raped by an intimate partner in the past 12 months. Most of these women present in emergency departments. Intimate violence can often result in traumatic stress, and stressful life-course events, such as menopause, retirement, loss of loved ones, onset of illness, and hospitalization, can worsen posttraumatic stress syndrome.[10]

In a 2009 study, Svavarsdottir and Orlygsdottie[11] assessed for serious emotional and physical health concerns among 2043 women in Massachusetts between 18 and 59 years of age who reported being abused by an intimate partner a year before the study. These investigators found that these women had chronic health conditions or illnesses, such as depression, fibromyalgia, fertility problems, and eating disorders. The women also smoked and misused alcohol. The authors supported interventions designed to decrease these health risk behaviors, treat chronic health conditions and illnesses, and offer first response to women who are victims of intimate partner violence to reduce the short- and long-term effects of violence on their physical and psychological heath. These investigators believe that public health nurses must focus specifically on intimate partner violence against women and that these professionals can play a leadership role in early identification and institution of appropriate interventions within primary health care settings.

A cross-sectional study by Ahmed and McCaw[12] from 2004 through 2009 found that 37% of women who experienced intimate violence used mental health services. The strongest predictor of use was electronic referral. Odds of use of mental health services were lower among Blacks, Latina, and Spanish-speaking patients. Patients who had experienced prior posttraumatic stress disorder or depression were more likely to use mental health services.

Another group of women who often experience intimate violence are those living with disabilities. A study in Canada in 2009 found that women who had physical, hearing, visual, learning, and mental health disabilities experienced not only intimate relation abuse but also abuse in health care settings, institutions, and in the home by a personal assistant. Three major recommendations came out of this study. The investigators determined that many women with disabilities do not have access to information relating to abuse prevention that is relevant culturally and linguistically, and therefore funds and resources should dedicated for organizations to provide accommodations, for example sign language interpretation or attendant services. The authors also recommended providing training in organizations that may come in contact with women with disabilities. Finally, they recommended universal screening, especially for rehabilitation providers.[13]

A study performed in rural health clinics between 2002 and 2005 concluded that a simple screening technique used during a physical can help identify women experiencing partner violence. Most of the 3664 women who were screened experienced IPV. Although 65.6% experienced both psychological battering and assault in their current relationships, 10.1% experienced assault only, and 24.3% experienced psychological battering only.[14] The screening technique used was the Women's Experience with Battering (WEB) Scale. The WEB scale measures psychological battering, and physical and sexual abuse in both their current and most recent relationship. Two items assess battering in past relationships. The authors recommend clinic-based IPV screening.[14]

The CDC has an extensive Web site related to IPV at http://www.cdc.gov/ViolencePrevention/intimatepartnerviolence/resources.html. An informative Web site about domestic violence is also available at http://www.thehotline.org/get-educated/what-is-domestic-violence.

Many states have a Domestic Violence Procedure Manuals that review responsibilities of the police and court systems.[15]

Although many agencies seem to exist that deal with intimate violence, no consistency seems to exist across disciplines. Procedures seem to vary among states. The 1994 Violence Against Women Act in the United States resulted in an estimated net benefit of $16.4 billion in averted victims' costs. This legislation introduced programs aimed at deterring crimes against women and provided assistance to female victims of crimes. Interventions include penalties for repeat offenders, use of sexual history in criminal and civil cases, and safe homes for women. A 2001 analysis shows that providing shelters for victims of domestic violence results in an estimated cost-benefit ratio of 18.4 to 6.8.[16]

Elderly

The debate in the field of elder abuse regarding whether elder abuse is caused by caregiver stress or abuser impairment has precipitated a discussion as to whether elder abuse should be a social service issue or a criminal justice problem. Even when family violence rises to the level of a crime as defined by state penal code, some professionals argue that a social service approach is best suited to address this social problem. A study by Brownell and Wolden[17] in 2002 used a nonexperimental study design to compare elder abuse situations served by Walk the Walk STEPS (Services to Empower and Protect Seniors) Crime Victims Programs with those served by the STEPS Elder Services Program. The investigators included sociodemographic profiles of the victims and abusers, types and circumstances of abuse, service interventions, and service outcomes. Walk the Walk has been in operation since 1997. Approximately 700 cases have been seen since the STEPS program started, with a current active caseload of 300. The results indicate that a social service intervention is more effective in achieving victim safety. It shows the importance of social service interventions in working with elder victims of crime. Graduate schools of social work should integrate aging and elder abuse content into the social work curriculum.

In 2004 Nelson and colleagues[18] examined evidence on the benefits and harms of screening women and elderly adults in health care settings for family violence and IPV. They found that no studies exist on the effectiveness of screening in a health care setting to reduce harm. Although literature regarding family violence and IPV is extensive, few studies provide data or detection and management standards to guide clinicians.[18]

The National Center on Elder Abuse (NCEA), directed by the U.S. Administration on Aging, is committed to helping national, state, and local partners in the field be fully prepared to ensure that older Americans live with dignity, integrity, independence, and without abuse, neglect, and exploitation. The NCEA is a resource for policy makers, social services and health care practitioners, the justice system, researchers, advocates, and families, and provides an information line for anyone suspecting elder abuse (800-677-1116).[19] The NCEA is another wonderful resource concerned with the prevalence and incidence of elder abuse. They have fact sheets and current statistics available for review.[19]

Prevention Strategies

Several strategies are recommended for prevention of interpersonal violence. The first is increasing the capacity for collecting and managing data. More support should be provided for research. Another important step is to promote primary prevention; systematic documentation of existing prevention programs should occur. The WHO has outlined a methodology for this documentation.[20] Support services for victims must be strengthened. Ready access to legal resources empowers victims. A national action plan for preventing interpersonal violence and improving support and care is the blueprint that will provide a set of common goals, a shared time frame, a strategy for coordinating activities, and a framework for evaluating different sectors involved. Collaboration among national governments and health-related nongovernmental and multilateral organizations can establish the importance of formally addressing violence through public health approaches.[20]

REFERENCES

1. World Health Organization (WHO). Interpersonal violence and alcohol policy briefing health priority. Geneva (Switzerland): WHO; 2005.

2. Recognizing child abuse and neglect: Signs and symptoms. Child Welfare Information Gateway; 2007. Available at: http://childwelfare.gov. Accessed May 3, 2011.
3. Schnitzer PG, Covington TM, Wirtz SJ, et al. Public health surveillance of fatal child maltreatment: analysis of 3 state programs. Am J Public Health 2008;98: 296–303.
4. Chartlier MJ, Walker JR, Nalmark B. Health risk behaviors and mental health problems as mediators of the relationship between childhood abuse and adult health. Am J Public Health 2009;99:847–54.
5. Prinz JP, Sanders MR, Shapiro CJ, et al. Population-based prevention of child maltreatment: the U.S. triple P system population trial. Prev Sci 2009;10:1–12.
6. Huebner CE. Evaluation of a clinic-based parent education program to reduce the risk of infant and toddler maltreatment. Public Health Nurs 2002;19:377–89.
7. U.S. Department of Health and Human Services, Administrative for Children and Families, Administration on Children, Youth and families Children's Bureau Child Welfare Information Gateway 2009. Available at: www.childwelfare.gov/pubs/reslist/tollfree.cfm. Accessed April 20, 2011.
8. State of New Jersey/Department of Children and Families. About the Division of Youth and Family Services 2011: Available at: www.state.nj.us/dcf/divisions/dyfs. Accessed April 20, 2011.
9. Thomas KA, Sorenson SB, Joshi M. Police documented incidents of intimate partner violence among young women. J Womens Health (Larchmt) 2010;19: 1079–87.
10. Sormanti M, Shibusawa T. Intimate partner violence among midlife and older women: a descriptive analysis of women seeking medical care. Health Soc Work 2008;933:33–41.
11. Svavarsdottir EK, Orlygsdottie B. Intimate Partner abuse factors associated with women's health: a general population study. J Adv Nurs 2009;65:1452–62.
12. Ahmed AT, McCaw BR. Mental health services utilization among women experiencing intimate partner violence. Am J Manag Care 2010;16:731–9.
13. Yoshida KK, Odette F, Hardie S, et al. Women living with disabilities and their experiences and issues related to the context and complexities of leaving abusive situations. Disabil Rehabil 2009;31:1843–52.
14. Coker AL, Flerx VC, Smith PH, et al. Partner violence screening in rural health care clinics. Am J Public Health 2007;97:1319–25.
15. State of New Jersey Domestic Violence Procedure Manual, October 2008. Available at: http://www.judiciary.state.nj.us/family/dvprcman.pdf. Accessed May 5, 2011.
16. Clark KA, Biddle AK, Martin SL. A cost-benefit analysis of the violence against women act of 1994 published erratum appears. Violence Against Women 2002; 8(4):417–28.
17. Brownell P, Wolden A. Elder abuse intervention strategies: social service or criminal justice? Journal of Gerontological Social Work 2002;40:83–100.
18. Nelson HD, Nygren P, McInerney Y, et al. Screening women and elderly adults for family and intimate partner violence: a review of the evidence for the US Preventative Services Task Force. Ann Intern Med 2004;1400:387–405.
19. National Center on Elder Abuse. NCEA Invites You to "Join Us in the Fight Against Elder Abuse." Available at: http://www.ncea.aoa.gov/NCEAroot/Main_Site/About/Initiatives/Join_Us_Campaign.aspx. Accessed May 5, 2011.
20. Sethi D, Marais M, Seedat J, et al. Handbook for the documentation of interpersonal violence prevention programs. Geneva (Switzerland): World health Organization, Department of Injuries and Violence Prevention; 2004.

Domestic and Institutional Elder Abuse Legislation

Jeanette M. Daly, RN, PhD

KEYWORDS

- Elder abuse • Adult protective services • Legislation • Statutes

Law is an important public health tool that plays a critical role for persons at risk for and victims of elder abuse. As of 1993, all 50 states and the District of Columbia had enacted legislation authorizing the provision of adult protective services (APS) in cases of elder abuse. North Carolina was the first state to enact a law in 1974, and New Jersey was the last in 1993.[1] The Older Americans Act[2] was the first federal law enacted to provide comprehensive services for older adults. It created the Administration on Aging and provided definitions of elder abuse. In March 2010, the first federal law directed at elder abuse was enacted, The Elder Justice Act (S.795).

The Elder Justice Act's main provisions include (1) establishment of an Elder Justice Coordinating Council to make recommendations on the coordination of federal, state, local, and private agencies related to elder abuse, (2) establishment of an advisory board to develop a strategic plan for developing the field of elder justice, (3) provision of APS funding, (4) establishment and support of forensic centers, (5) provision of long-term care ombudsman program funding, (6) provision of grants to enhance long-term care staffing, (7) provision of funding for a national training institute for surveyors, and (8) provision of funding for a national nurse aide registry. In addition, it requires immediate reporting of crimes in long-term care facilities, and imposes penalties for retaliation against an employee who filed a complaint and for failure to report.

Legislation has different meanings, such as a bill or statutory law. When an item is being written and considered for a law, it is known as a *bill*. Once the bill is enacted it is a *statute*. Statutes are laws passed by the United States Congress or a state legislature. Regulations are generated after statutes to outline how these statutes will be enforced. Legislative bodies write statutory law, whereas administrative agencies of the executive branch of government produce regulations. Statutes and regulations are written by all levels of government—federal, state, and local—and are generally published in two versions: a chronologic version and a codified version.

The author has nothing to disclose.
Department of Family Medicine, Carver College of Medicine, University of Iowa, 01290-F PFP, 200 Hawkins Drive, Iowa City, IA 52242, USA
E-mail address: jeanette-daly@uiowa.edu

TYPES OF ELDER ABUSE LEGISLATION

State laws that have been enacted to protect older persons vary, including the implementation of protective service programs, licensing and recertification laws for institutions and facilities, the enabling laws of the federal Older Americans Act and long-term care ombudsman program, laws pertaining to Medicaid fraud, and laws requiring criminal prosecution of certain types of elder abuse.[1] Legislation for elder abuse in the domestic setting is usually found in APS-related laws. Legislation regarding licensure and recertification and long-term care ombudsman programs provides laws for elder abuse in institutional settings. However, many state laws provide for domestic and institutional settings; each state is unique.

The APS-related laws were enacted primarily to control elder abuse in the domestic or institutional setting, depending on the state. Generally, these APS laws establish a system for the reporting and investigation of elder abuse and the provision of social services to help victims and ameliorate the abuse. In most states, these laws pertain to abused adults who have a disability, vulnerability, or impairment as defined by state law, not just to older persons. Some states, however, have distinct elder protective services laws or programs. An example of a policy statement about this type of law is from Nevada: "It is the policy of this State to provide for the cooperation of law enforcement officials, courts of competent jurisdiction and all appropriate state agencies providing human services in identifying the abuse, neglect, exploitation and isolation of older persons and vulnerable persons through the complete reporting of abuse, neglect, exploitation and isolation of older persons and vulnerable persons."[3]

Procedures for investigating complaints in nursing homes classified as nursing facilities or skilled nursing facilities are established by each state's respective legislation and a minimal set of standards established by the Federal Nursing Home Reform Act.[4] Through the licensure and recertification legislation, provisions are implemented for the development, establishment, and enforcement of basic standards for the health, care, and treatment of persons in nursing homes and for the maintenance and operation of these institutions. An example of a purpose statement about this type of law is from Illinois: "The Illinois Department of Public Health shall upon receiving reports made under this Act, seek to protect residents and prevent further harm to the resident who was the subject of the report and other residents in the facility. In performing these duties, the Department may utilize such protective services of other State departments, commissions, boards or other agencies and any voluntary agencies as are available."[5]

The long-term care ombudsman program provides advocacy for residents of nursing homes, board and care homes, and assisted living, and is administered by the Administration on Aging.[6,7] Ombudsmen offer information to the public about facilities and how to obtain quality of care.[8,9] Part of their mission is to resolve problems and assist residents with complaints. Permission from the resident must be provided for an ombudsman to share complaints with other agency staff.[8,9] Nursing home complaints to ombudsmen have increased from 145,000 in 1996 to 271,000 in 2008.[8] An example of a purpose statement for this type of law is from Maine: "In accordance with the program established…the ombudsman may enter onto the premises of any [licensed] residential care facility…, any assisted living facility…and any nursing facility to investigate complaints concerning those facilities or to perform any other functions authorized by this section or other applicable law or rules."[10]

Elder Abuse Legislation Research

Research conducted regarding elder abuse legislation is scarce. Through 2008, 23 journal publications were found from 16 health care and criminal justice literature databases on abuse of persons aged 55 years and older in the United States.[11] Early research described the content of the few state statutes that had legislation for mandatory reporting of adult abuse,[12] the impact of mandatory reporting on the victim,[13] the rights and restrictions of nurses regarding mandatory reporting,[14] and the change in reporting of elder abuse cases after implementation of mandatory reporting.[15] An overview of content covering elder abuse[16,17] and definitions of elder abuse[18] in APS-related statutes were given, and an overview of content of certification and relicensure statutes covering institutional elder abuse[19] and statute definitions of elder abuse[20] was provided.

Surveys regarding elder abuse legislation have explored perceived effectiveness of legislation by social workers,[21] health department administrators' knowledge of the elder abuse law,[22] and public attitudes toward the definition and criminalization of elder abuse over a 10-year period.[23] Perceptions of police chiefs and ombudsmen were compared regarding the seriousness of elder abuse incidents and the role of criminal penalties.[24] Physicians' knowledge of elder abuse law and their willingness to report cases of elder abuse were explored, with findings indicating that only the most obvious and severe cases were reported.[25] A survey of all nursing home administrators and directors of nursing in Iowa found that those who indicated a greater knowledge of the elder abuse law worked at facilities with higher report rates of nursing home abuse.[26] Length of time in one's position, facility, and profession was negatively associated with report rates.[26] A complete statewide profile of the response by state authorities of reported abuse was described for older female victims of abuse.[27]

Other research conducted on the content of the law focuses on rates of elder abuse reports, investigations, and substantiations. This research is conducted by the same investigators, Daly and Jogerst.[28–33] In their work, a *report* is an allegation of abuse received by an investigating agency. An *investigation* is the process undertaken to evaluate the potential victim after a report has been filed. *Substantiation* is the finding that abuse actually exists according to state law.

A landmark study was conducted in 2003 evaluating the impact of state APS-related legislation on rates of elder abuse reports, investigations, and substantiations.[28] For this study, a compilation was made of the annual reports of APS agencies' numbers of elder abuse reports, investigations, and substantiations for each state and the District of Columbia. Statutes were retrieved and reviewed, and the content coded to determine the presence or absence of text addressing items such as recording a report of abuse, mandatory reporting, definitions of abuse, penalty for failure to report abuse, dependent vulnerable person covered by statute, and education for caseworkers. Key findings from this study included:

- Higher reported rates of abuse correlated with states requiring public education regarding elder abuse, suggesting that increased public awareness increases reporting of elder abuse.
- States that have the requirement of mandatory reporting had a significantly higher investigation rate.
- Thirty-three states had a provision for penalties for failure to report abuse, and this also was significantly associated with higher investigation rates.
- Investigation rates were almost identical among states with and without the criterion of adult dependence or vulnerability.
- Higher numbers of abuse definitions in the regulations were associated with higher substantiation rates.
- A state's administrative decision to track reports of abuse led to significantly higher investigation and substantiation rates.

- A higher proportion of total population categorized as elderly was associated with lower substantiation rates.

Continuing this work with a specific focus on mandatory reporting, the purpose of the next study was to evaluate the relationship between the wording of state APS-related mandatory reporting legislation and the rates of reported, investigated, and substantiated domestic elder abuse.[29] The same data were used as in the earlier study, and the research team found the following:

- Six states do not regulate mandatory reporters (Colorado, New Jersey, New York, North Dakota, South Dakota, and Wisconsin).
- Higher investigation rates were associated with a mandatory reporting requirement.
- Penalty for failure to report abuse allegations did not result in a significant difference in report, investigation, and substantiation rates.
- The substance of how the mandatory reporting requirement was written in the statute (ie, listing all the mandatory reporters or just saying "any person") was not important.
- Time to report an abuse allegation, such as within 24 hours or within 1 week, did not result in a significant difference in report, investigation, and substantiation rates.
- Health care professionals and law enforcement personnel are frequently listed as mandatory reporters.
- Education of mandatory reporters is required only by Iowa law.

Focusing on the fact that Iowa is the only state with a law that requires education for its mandatory reporters of elder abuse, another study was conducted. Its purpose was to compare the investigation and substantiation rates for elder abuse allegations before and after July 1988, when Iowa statute[30] was revised to ensure training of mandatory reporters, and to determine whether required education increases reporting and substantiation rates.[31] A comparison of the time periods showed no significant differences in investigation or substantiation rates, indicating that education has not impacted the number of cases of elder abuse.

Again using the original data from the first study, the research team, with social work graduate students, explored the relationship between required educational background of APS workers and the rates of reported, investigated, and substantiated domestic elder abuse.[32] If the statutes did not include the information, additional information was gathered from APS administrators regarding education of elder abuse APS workers,. The main finding was that no educational or licensure requirements for APS workers were identified in the statutes. Regulations for seven states and the District of Columbia required a baccalaureate degree, and four states and the District of Columbia required that degree to be in social work. Findings indicated no significant differences in report, investigation, and substantiation rates among states that have regulations that require a baccalaureate degree or social work license and those that do not. However, investigation rates were significantly higher for states that have regulations requiring a social work degree compared with those that do not.

Expanding the original data set to include specific penalties in the law, another study was conducted to evaluate the impact of criminal penalties for the infliction of abuse on the rates of reported, investigated, and substantiated domestic elder abuse for all states.[33] Penalties were designated in the statutes as felonies or misdemeanors and might include fines or imprisonment. If the APS-related statutes did not indicate one particular penalty, then the state's statute prescribing criminal penalties for each offense category was reviewed. Significant findings are listed below:

- Forty-three states and the District of Columbia categorize elder abuse as a felony and prescribe imprisonment for the act.
- Thirty states regard elder abuse as a misdemeanor and prescribe fines and/or imprisonment.
- Twenty-four states have both felonies and misdemeanors for various types of abuse.
- Thirty-nine states prescribe fines for felonies.
- Felony fines range from $500 to $1 million, with a mean of $51,700.
- Prison terms for a felony ranged from 1.5 to 99 years, with a mean of 14 years.
- A significant positive association was seen between having felony fines and higher substantiation rates.

Taking a political viewpoint, the research team conducted a study detailing the types of and motivations for state elder abuse law, including interpretive regulations and legislation.[34] This study describes the rationale behind different states' elder abuse laws and regulations, and why the way they were written influences the investigation and substantiation of domestic elder abuse. Variables analyzed included political, structural, and socioeconomic measures, such as word count, number of definitions in the regulations, and joint investigation of elder and child abuse. Findings indicated that legislator characteristics (being middle-aged or slightly older) and lobbying by important interest groups have an unexpected effect, suggesting that issues exist that seem more pressing than elder abuse.

Focusing on institutional elder abuse, another study was conducted to identify state and nursing home characteristics associated with the rates of nursing home resident mistreatment.[35] A national data set, the federal complaint/incident system, was used to discern factors influencing nursing home abuse. Content of the law had an impact on rates of nursing home abuse, and states that have statutes requiring the facility, rather than an individual, to report mistreatment had lower incidents. Higher complaints were significantly associated with lower levels of staffing.

Variations in Elder Abuse Legislation

Variations by state in the statutes and regulations lead to noticeable differences in the implementation of the law. These differences begin with the state agency assigned to administer the adult protective service component. The program may be state-administered or county-administered. The program itself may include the investigation of both child and elder abuse reports, or these investigations may be assigned to separate agencies. Organizational structure for each state is different for domestic and institutional abuse reporting. For example, Alabama's responsible APS agency is the Department of Human Resources, whereas it is the Department of Health and Human Services for California, the Department of Aging in Illinois, and Family and Social Services Administration in Indiana. For licensure and recertification investigating agencies, the organizational structure is also different according to state. In Iowa, it is the Department of Inspections and Appeals, whereas in Maryland it is the Office of Health Care Quality.

Statute definitions of elder mistreatment are not identical but have common threads. No one definition of elder abuse encompasses all varieties of mistreatment.[36] Common elements in statute definitions are abuse, neglect, and exploitation. Variations then occur within the common elements, such as neglect, self-neglect, and abuse defined as physical, sexual, emotional, or psychological. Investigating agencies must apply the state-specific definition in their investigations.

Statute language that defines persons who are dependent or vulnerable regarding elder abuse is extremely diverse.[37,38] For example, 12 states use the term *vulnerable adult* as the primary concept title, 6 states use the terms *elderly person* or *adult*, 5 states use the term *disabled person*, 4 states use the terms *dependent adult* and *in need of protective services*, 4 states use the terms *older person*, *endangered adult*, *at-risk adult*, and *eligible adult*, and 1 state uses the terms *elderly adult*, *infirm adult*, *impaired adult*, and *incapacitated adult*. One state, Rhode Island, did not have a definition.[1]

Another difference in the legislative definition of the vulnerable adult is the inclusion or exclusion of age of the dependent/vulnerable adult. Nine states do not include an age range in their adult protective service law, whereas 18 designate the range as 18 years of age or older, 12 use 60 years of age or older, and 3 use 65 years of age or older in their respective laws.[1]

In the licensure and recertification statutes, only 14 states have statutes with text specifically addressing the topic of abuse reports and investigation in nursing homes.[19] Thus, the most states do not have statute text addressing nursing home abuse investigations.

Among these 14 states, 10 statutes list 22 different types of abuse, including chemical restraint, confinement, financial exploitation, neglect, physical restraint, and sexual abuse.[19] Physical abuse and neglect were types of mistreatment listed in all 14 statutes relating to nursing homes.[20] However, types of nursing home abuse were not listed in the other licensure and recertification statutes.

The investigation process of the alleged abuse is described for 12 of 50 states, some in detail and others minimally. For example, Georgia's detailed investigation text reads:

The department shall immediately initiate an investigation after the receipt of any report. The department shall direct and conduct all investigations; however, it may delegate the conduct of investigations to local police authorities or other appropriate agencies. If such delegation occurs, the agency to which authority has been delegated must report the results of its investigation to the department immediately upon completion. The investigation shall determine the nature, cause, and extent of the reported abuse or exploitation, an assessment of the current condition of the resident, and an assessment of needed action and services. Where appropriate, the investigation shall include a prompt visit to the resident.[39]

However, New Hampshire's statute provides minimal detail about investigation: "the attorney general shall be responsible for the investigation and prosecution of patient abuse or neglect in any health care facility, whether licensed or unlicensed."[19,40]

Statutes pertinent to elder abuse vary widely. This article provides examples of organizational structure, dependency and age of the victim, definitions of abuse, classification of penalties, and investigation processes. Health care providers must learn their state's elder abuse laws and review any operating manuals produced from the statutes or regulations. All health care workers must know and implement the law to protect the welfare of older persons. As noted in *The Future of the Public's Health in the 21st Century*, "public health law at the federal, state and local levels is often outdated and internally inconsistent...."[41] It is ultimately important to take responsibility and help change the laws to conform to modern scientific and legal standards.

REFERENCES

1. Tatara T. An analysis of state laws addressing elder abuse, neglect, and exploitation. Washington, DC: National Center on Elder Abuse; 1995.
2. Pub.L. 89–73, 79 Stat. 218, July 14, 1965.
3. Nev. Rev. Stat. Ann. §200.5091.
4. National Long-Term Care Ombudsman Resource Center. What does an ombudsman do? Available at: http://www.ltcombudsman.org/about-ombudsmen. Accessed February 21, 2011.
5. 210 Ill. Comp. Stat. Ann. 30/2 from Ch. 1111 1/2, par. 4162.
6. Netting FE, Huber R, Paton RN, et al. Elder rights and the long-term care ombudsman program. Soc Work 1995;40(3):351–7.
7. Price DM. The ombudsman experience: administrative protection for vulnerable patients. Trends Health Care Law Ethics 2003;8(1):49–56.
8. National long term care ombudsman resource center. (2001). OBRA '87. Retrieved February 2, 2007 from. Available at: http://www.ltcombudsman.org/ombpublic/49_346_1023.cfm. Accessed February 2, 2007.
9. Schneider DC, Mosqueda L, Falk E, et al. Elder abuse forensic centers. J Elder Abuse Negl 2010;22(3–4):255–74.
10. ME. Rev. Stat. Ann. Tit. 22 §5107-A.
11. Daly JM, Merchant GJ, Jogerst GJ. Elder abuse research: a systematic review. J Elder Abuse Negl 2011, in press.
12. Salend E, Kane RA, Satz M, et al. Elder abuse reporting: limitations of statutes. Gerontologist 1984;24(1):61–7.
13. Rodriguez MA, Wallace SP, Woolf NH, et al. Mandatory reporting of elder abuse: between a rock and a hard place. Ann Fam Med 2006;4(5):403–9.
14. Thobaben M, Anderson L. Reporting elder abuse: it's the law. Am J Nurs 1985; 85(4):371–4.
15. Fredriksen KI. Adult protective services: changes with the introduction of mandatory reporting. J Elder Abuse Negl 1989;1(2):59–70.
16. Capezuti E, Brush BL, Lawson WT III. Reporting elder mistreatment. J Gerontol Nurs 1997;23(7):24–32.
17. Roby JL, Sullivan R. Adult protection service laws: a comparison of state statutes from definition to case closure. J Elder Abuse Negl 2000;12(3/4):17–51.
18. Daly JM, Jogerst GJ. Statute definitions of elder abuse. J Elder Abuse Negl 2001; 13(4):39–57.
19. Daly J, Jogerst G. Nursing home abuse report and investigation legislation. J Elder Abuse Negl 2007;19(3–4):119–31.
20. Daly JM, Jogerst GJ. Nursing home statutes: mistreatment definitions. J Elder Abuse Negl 2006;18(1):19–39.
21. Bond JB, Penner RL. Perceived effectiveness of legislation concerning abuse of the elderly: a survey of professionals in Canada and the United States. Can J Aging 1995;14(Suppl 2):118–35.
22. Ehrlich P, Anetzberger G. Survey of state public health departments on procedures for reporting elder abuse. Public Health Rep 1991;106(2):151–4.
23. Morgan E, Johnson I, Sigler R. Public definitions and endorsement of the criminalization of elder abuse. J Crim Justice 2006;34:275–83.
24. Payne BK, Berg BL. Perceptions about the criminalization of elder abuse among police chiefs and ombudsmen. Crime Delinq 2003;49(3):439–59.
25. Clark-Daniels CL, Baumhover LA, Daniels RS. To report or not to report: Physicians' response to elder abuse. J Health Hum Resour Adm 1990;13(1):52–70.

26. Daly JM, Jogerst GJ. Association of knowledge of adult protective services legislation with rates of reporting of abuse in Iowa nursing homes. J Am Med Dir Assoc 2005;6(2):113–20.
27. Klein A, Tobin T, Salomon A, et al. A statewide profile of abuse of older women and the criminal justice response. Sudbury (MA): Advocates for Human Potential, Inc; 2008.
28. Jogerst G, Daly JM, Brinig M, et al. Domestic elder abuse and the law. Am J Public Health 2003;93(12):2131–6.
29. Daly JM, Jogerst GJ, Brinig M, et al. Mandatory reporting: relationship of APS statute language on state reported elder abuse. J Elder Abuse Negl 2003; 15(2):1–21.
30. Iowa Code. § 235B.1.
31. Jogerst GJ, Daly JM, Dawson J, et al. Required education for Iowa mandatory reporters of elder abuse. J Elder Abuse Negl 2003;15(1):59–73.
32. Daly JM, Jogerst GJ, Haigh KM, et al. APS workers job requirements affecting elder abuse rates. Soc Work Health Care 2005;40(3):89–102.
33. Jogerst GJ, Daly JM, Brinig MF, et al. The association between statutory penalties and domestic elder abuse investigations. J Crim Justice 2005;28(2):52–69.
34. Brinig MF, Jogerst GJ, Daly JM, et al. Public choice and domestic elder abuse law. J Leg Stud 2004;33(2):517–49.
35. Jogerst GJ, Daly JM, Hartz AJ. State policies and nursing home characteristics associated with rates of resident mistreatment. J Am Med Dir Assoc 2008;9: 648–56.
36. Moskowitz S. Saving granny from the wolf: elder abuse and neglect - the legal framework. Conn Law Rev 1998;31(77):204.
37. Hall GR, Weiler K. Elder abuse, neglect, and mistreatment. In: Bradway CW, editor. Nursing care of geriatric emergencies. New York: Springer Publishing company, Inc; 1996. p. 225–51.
38. National Center on Elder Abuse. "Vulnerable Adult" definitions discussed on abuse listserve. Newsletter National Center on Elder Abuse 1999;1(3):2.
39. Official Code of Georgia Annotated. §31-8-83.
40. New Hampshire Revised Statutes Annotated. §151:27.
41. National Academy of Sciences. The future of the public's health in the 21st century. Washington, DC: The National Academies Press; 2003.

Meeting the 2015 Millennium Development Goals with New Interventions for Abused Women

Rozina Karmaliani, PhD, RN[a],*, Shireen Shehzad, BScN[b],
Saima Shams Hirani, MSN, RN[b], Nargis Asad, PhD[c],
Shela Akbar Ali Hirani, MSN[b], Judith McFarlane, DrPH, RN[d]

KEYWORDS

• Millennium developmental goals 2015 • Interventions
• Abused women • Pakistan

The Millennium Development Goals (MDGs) 2015 were adopted in September 2000 by the United Nations' Development Program.[1] The declaration recognizes the need for global attention to critical issues to maximize world health. In order of priority, the MDGs include: eradication of extreme poverty and hunger; achievement of universal primary education; promotion of gender equality and empowerment of women; reduction in child mortality; improvement of maternal health; combating of HIV/AIDS, malaria, and other diseases; ensuring of environmental sustainability; and development of global partnerships for development.

This research is supported by Grant No. ID: 072020RAD from Aga Khan University Research Council.
The authors have nothing to disclose.
[a] School of Nursing and Department of Community Health Sciences, Aga Khan University, P.O. Box# 3500, Stadium Road, Karachi 74800, Pakistan
[b] School of Nursing, Aga Khan University, PO Box #3500, Stadium Road, Karachi 74800, Pakistan
[c] Department of Psychiatry, The Aga Khan University Hospital, Faculty Offices Building, Karachi 74800, Pakistan
[d] Texas Woman's University, Nelda C. Stark College of Nursing, Houston Center, 6700 Fannin Street, Houston, TX 77030, USA
* Corresponding author.
E-mail address: rozina.karmaliani@aku.edu

Nurs Clin N Am 46 (2011) 485–493
doi:10.1016/j.cnur.2011.08.002
0029-6465/11/$ – see front matter © 2011 Elsevier Inc. All rights reserved.

Pakistan, one of the developing countries of South Asia, is a low-income country with around 172 million inhabitants with major segments of the population deprived of education, access to health care, and basic housing.[2] Some two-thirds of the Pakistani population exists on less than one United States dollar a day. Therefore, evidence-based, culturally sensitive, and community-applicable interventions are essential to meet the MDGs and decrease the obstacles of illiteracy, poverty, poor health, and gender inequities that result in abuse against women.

Pakistan is a male dominated society where abuse of women by the males is an accepted norm. Women in Pakistan report high levels of physical and sexual abuse from their intimate partners and many abused women consider the violence an inevitable part of their lives.[3] Like women worldwide, women in Pakistan undergo violence at various stages in their life, including during pregnancy. Although research in this regard is sparse, past research in Pakistan with pregnant women has documented that 18% of the pregnant women had anxiety and/or depression, with physical or sexual and verbal abuse during pregnancy—the most common risk factor for poor mental health.[4] Similarly, suicidal thoughts and attempts in the pregnant cohort were estimated to be quite high; 11% of the women studied had considered suicide and 45% had attempted suicide. Women who had anxiety or depression, or had experienced verbal, physical, or sexual abuse were significantly more likely to have had suicidal thoughts and to have attempted suicide.[5]

In the global context of violence against women, Pakistani statistics are appreciably high for life-time exposure to physical and sexual violence. In a recent report, figures reported for physical and sexual abuse are 57.6% and 54.5%, respectively, among a sample of 759 women in a community-based cross-sectional study.[2]

Poor women in Pakistan are usually not paid for their hours of toil and have no income and very little to no say in family matters.[2] External to the domestic abuse that confronts multitudes of women daily in Pakistan; multiethnic civil disturbances are common in the country. Hence, it is common for women to be sequestered in their homes for days due to terrorist threats and actual attacks, homicides, and ethnic-political warfare that derails women's economic empowerment and employment, which is linked to household income and directly tied to nutrition and health of women and children, as cited in the 2015 MDGs.[1]

MEETING THE MDGS WITH NEW INTERVENTIONS FOR ABUSED WOMEN

Better health for women and children is essential to achieve the MDGs. Regarding women's health issues, a literature review that documents the epidemic global health burden of mental disorders shows that women are twice as likely to have depression as men.[6,7] There are various reasons for higher rates of depression among women. Depression and partner violence coexist for many women.[8,9] Children of depressed mothers have a variety of developmental, behavioral, and mental health problems compared with children whose mothers are not depressed.[10,11] Research evidence documents that low socioeconomic status is consistently associated with a higher prevalence of depression.[12] Frequently, the partner violence and accompanying depression begin during pregnancy.[13] Results from a recent study in Pakistan show that verbal and physical abuse during pregnancy is the most significant predictor of depression and anxiety among urban women.[14] Children who witness partner violence or whose mothers are victimized by violence have appreciable problems with social skills, learning, depression, and aggression.[15,16] However, research shows that providing treatment to the abused and depressed mother can improve the functioning of the children in just 6 months.[17,18]

The World Health Report (WHO), "Make Every Mother and Child Count,"[19] stresses an urgent need for community-based programs that offer counseling, support, and information.

In Southern Asia, the urgency to derive and test new interventions to decrease abuse of women is further accentuated because women are far more affected by poverty, illiteracy, and unemployment compared with men.[1] The largest share (some 46%) of women's employment is as contributing family workers (eg, managing the family market stall, cooking for the family restaurant). These women, also known as unpaid family workers, add to the heavy burden of unpaid work done by women in households in Pakistan.

With the goal of forming and testing new strategies for abused women living in poor communities of Karachi, Pakistan, a multidisciplinary research team comprised of clinical psychologist and nurses, working across various disciplines of nursing, community health sciences, and pediatrics, selected two interventions for field testing in a randomized clinical trial. The first intervention was a counseling model, previously empirically tested with good results in Pakistan.[20] The second intervention, economic skill building, was conceptually and operationally derived by the research team following focus group discussions with community leaders.[4,21] The team tested the differential effectiveness of economic skill building and counseling on the mental health, reported abuse, and self-efficacy outcomes of women, and the behavioral functioning of their children.

The goal of the authors' research was to address the primary health problems confronting women worldwide (ie, depression and violence) and, simultaneously, to enhance the psychological health of children. The two community-based interventions were tested with mothers who were enrolled in a literacy program and who had at least one child between the ages of 18 months and 16 years. The strategy of enrolling women from the adult literacy classes was used for recruitment of all the three groups: two intervention groups and one control group. Hence, all women participated in an adult literacy class daily for 1 hour, for a total of 5 hours per week. Both intervention groups received an additional hour once a week for the intervention: counseling or economic skill building. The control group only received the Adult Literacy Program.

The approach was straightforward. A mentally healthy mother is better able to care for herself and her children. The hypothesis was that with improved maternal mental health the entire family would be less stressed and able to obtain better family cohesion and higher functioning. The essential components of each intervention are discussed, followed by the women's reactions to the interventions. Finally, the next step is presented: the test of a microlending intervention to improve women's health, based on the women's recommendations and MDGs goals.

Group Counseling: Intervention One

Acknowledging the epidemic global health burden of women being twice more likely than men to have depression,[22] one of the interventions selected was group counseling. Throughout their childbearing years, women experience significantly higher rates of depression than men. The female-to-male ratio is approximately two to one.[23] Pakistan reports one of the highest rates for psychiatric morbidity in the world, with 66% of women depressed.[24]

Group counseling is well recognized as a cost-effective approach to meeting mental health needs. Group counseling, as opposed to treatment as usual, has shown favorable results in resource-deprived communities.[25]

Previous research in Pakistan using Lady Health Workers to offer basic mental health services to women, demonstrated positive results. Using a tested and effective counselor-led training model, Lady Health Workers from an economically deprived community were trained, using the counseling training manual as set forth by Ali and Rahber,[20] but with a group process approach, that enabled the project to be sensitive to cultural diversity and women's safety, and to offer mental health services to many women.

Twelve hours of training was offered to the Lady Health Workers who would deliver the counseling. Training focused on empathetic listening, supportive communication skills, and systematic problem solving. Empathetic listening was taught through role-play and open discussions. Six groups of randomly assigned women, in groups of five to six, received the counseling intervention.

Economic Skills Building: Intervention Two

Association between women's mental health and domestic violence is well documented; however, the connections between better mental health, less abuse, and better health for women and children has not been researched to any great extent. Economic stability is considered one of the significant key determinants of health, yet being in an abusive relationship typically restricts women's economic independence, making employment difficult,[26–28] limiting access to income, and impeding women's self-efficacy after leaving the abuser.[29] The WHO[30] has endorsed this aspect; has identified economic resources as an important element for reducing violence against women; and has called for research that explores the casual association between economic inequality, weak safety nets, unemployment, and poverty.[31] Therefore, to address the MDGs for decreasing economic inequities, an economic skill building intervention was created and tested on women.

The economic skill building intervention, like the counseling intervention, was delivered through the trained community health workers for 8 weeks, one session per week, at the adult literacy centers. These women were also randomly assigned and completed the economic skill building training in groups of six to eight. The economic skill-building intervention was developed with the help of key informants from the community and a thorough literature review. It included skills for employment attainment and retention such as effective communication, balancing of personal and work life, time management, conflict resolution, dealing with abuse and harassment, enhancing self-efficacy, effective parenting, and personal hygiene and grooming.[21,32]

After 12 months of applying both the interventions, three focus group discussions were conducted: one for each intervention group and one for the control group. Twenty-five women attended the three focus groups: eight from the economic skill building group, seven from the counseling intervention, and ten from the control group. The purpose of the focus group discussions was to learn about the women's experiences and opinions regarding the two interventions of economic skill building and counseling, and the stand-alone adult literacy program.

The major themes derived were classified as Challenges Faced by Women, Outcomes Following the Interventions, and Recommendations.

Challenges Faced by Women

There were certain challenges shared during the focus group discussions that were faced by the women in all the three groups. All women considered control and resistance by their husbands and in-laws as a major barrier to pursuing self-efficacy and financial decision-making, further education, socialization with other women, and economic empowerment. The literature supports that restriction in women's participation in productive employment, women's access to education, and domestic violence are associated with poor effects on women's health and children's wellbeing.[33]

Additional constraints discussed by the economic skill building group focused on the job market and difficulty in obtaining jobs. The women discussed environmental safety issues, which precluded them from going to work without threat of bodily harm; age expectations; staying at home with children; marital and family responsibilities as prescribed by husband and in-laws; the parenting role expectation that only the mother could adequately care for the children; and the required skills and necessary education for employment opportunities.

Outcomes Following the Interventions

The women in all the three groups acknowledged the positive effects of the interventions that they received in addressing these challenges, including economic skill building, counseling, or stand-alone adult literacy. The women who had received the counseling intervention discussed positive changes in themselves, most commonly pertaining to their self-management of emotions, including anger management and improved communication with family members. One of the participants from the counseling group stated, "All the aggression in my nature is now settled and I feel much better and mature instead of being confused. Now our husbands know that we can utter our opinion."

The women who had received the economic skill building intervention also emphasized having attained more self-efficacy and self-management of feelings. The women further shared that they now had better self-awareness, more strength of character, hope for the future, and better problem-solving skills for improved marital and parent–child relationships. One woman expressed, "These sessions have worked a miracle for me as my daughter seems to enjoy the fact that I have transformed into a more understanding mother and I can deal with domestic matters without any trouble."

The women who had only received the stand-alone adult literacy program shared perceived self-improvement, primarily in the areas of reading and writing skills, "If a woman is educated herself then she can understand her children better."

RECOMMENDATIONS

The recommendations for further interventions, as suggested by the women, focused on developing strategies for establishing support groups for women and skill building to overcome barriers faced by women in obtaining and retaining employment. All women desired employment but thought they needed additional social and economic empowerment skills to be successful. All women mentioned the benefits of group socialization and focused work on communication and other life skills. As one woman verbalized, "It was great help for me in my daily life and it was a great feeling when I sat with you all and shared my feelings as I had no one to talk and share (at home)."

The researchers felt that, the women of all the three groups felt more empowered through group socialization. Significant improvements in self-efficacy were documented by earlier reports of the findings using a scored self-efficacy instrument.[32] Self-efficacy is considered a significant contributor toward women's positive mental health[34] and it can enable women to adapt successfully in distressful situations, such as domestic violence.[35,36] The findings agree with the WHO[22] document, regarding the importance of strategies to promote women economic empowerment to deal with sociocultural challenges, including abuse against women. Following the intervention trial findings[32] and focus group work with the women described herein, the authors' think a combination of further economic skill building interventions and revenue investment for starting small women-owned businesses has good potential for poverty alleviation and better mental health outcomes for women and their children in Pakistan.

The Road Ahead: Testing Microcredit for Better Health and Meeting MDGs

What is the next step to meet the MDGs and achieve better health and less abuse for poor women in Pakistan and worldwide? The association between wealth and health is well established. Poor people experience poor health. Women with children disproportionately represent the poor people of the world. When a woman is economically disadvantaged, her health suffers and the growth and development of her children are jeopardized. MDGs 2015 focus on eradicating extreme poverty and hunger by halving the proportion of persons whose income is less than a dollar a day.[1]

In a developing country such as Pakistan, where women face poor health and domestic violence related to lack of economic empowerment, microcredit is considered an antipoverty tool that can to empower women to achieve gender equity and better health.[37] Microcredit, also referred to as microfinance, fills a gap in many developing countries where cultural and social constraints limit opportunities for underserved communities.[38] Microfinance provides opportunities to residents of underserved communities, especially to women with limited or no access to traditional lending, to start small businesses, generate income, and progress toward self-sufficiency. Microfinance can connect economic empowerment interventions, such as economic skill building, with better health and achievement of the MDGs.[39–41]

The literature supports the finding that microfinance has a considerable impact on women's self-confidence, decision making, and empowerment; and it prepares women for addressing the inequality issues at the family and community level.[37,40,42] Microcredit programs report reductions in the incidences of men's violence against women by promoting economic and social independence of abused women in the society.[43] Research indicates the need to test the effectiveness of microcredit with, and without, economic skill building and counseling for the abused women in Pakistan.

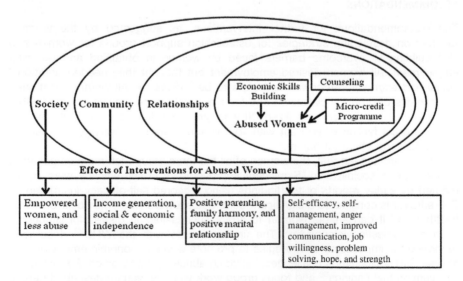

Fig. 1. An Ecological Model to study interventions for abused women.

The authors' identified no research that tested microcredit and its impact on women's health and children's wellbeing in Pakistan. To advance interventions for abused women, to work toward MDGs 2015, and to build on our research findings with economic skill building and counseling, our team has adopted an Ecological Model, as presented in **Fig. 1**, which is proposed by WHO[22] as a holistic model from which to study effective interventions for abused women. The model begins with the impact of the intervention on the individual abused woman and builds to the positive effect on the family, community, and society, including the potential attainment of better gender equity.

SUMMARY

The authors' believe that the best interventions for abused women are those derived from culturally sensitive partnerships with communities and those that are frequently enriched with the voices of the people. We embrace the ecological model proposed by WHO[22] as an optimum method to work toward ending of abuse of women and attainment of the MDGs 2015.

ACKNOWLEDGMENTS

The authors' gratefully acknowledge the community members, key informants, and focus group participants of Bilal Colony in Karachi, Pakistan for their participation. We thank the Aga Khan University Research Council (URC) and the Sindh Education Foundation (SEF) for their partnership toward adult literacy for women.

REFERENCES

1. The Millennium Development Goals Report, United Nation 2009. Available at: http://www.un.org/millenniumgoals/pdf/MDG%20Report%202009%20ENG.pdf. Accessed March 25, 2011.
2. Ali TS, Asad N, Mogren N, et al. Intimate partner violence in urban Pakistan: prevalence, frequency and risk factors. Int J Womens Health 2011;3:105–15.
3. Rabbani F, Quereshi F, Rizvi N. Perspectives on domestic violence: case study from Karachi, Pakistan. East Mediterr Health J 2008;14(2):412–26.
4. Karmaliani R, Asad N, Bann CM, et al. Prevalence of anxiety, depression, and associated factors among pregnant women of Hyderabad, Pakistan. Int J Soc Psychiatry 2009;55:414–24.
5. Asad N, Karmaliani R, Sulaiman N, et al. Prevalence of suicidal thoughts and attempts among pregnant Pakistani women. Acta Obstet Gynecol Scand 2010; 89(12):1545–51.
6. World Health Report. Women's mental health: an evidence based review. Geneva (Switzerland): World Health Organization; 2000.
7. World Health Report. Mental health: new understanding, new hope. Geneva (Switzerland): World Health Organization; 2001.
8. Nixon RD, Resick PA, Nishith P. An exploration of comorbid depression among female victims of intimate partner violence with posttraumatic stress disorder. J Affect Disord 2004;82:315–20.
9. Hegarty K, Gunn J, Chondros P, et al. Association between depression and abuse by partners of women attending general practice: descriptive, cross-sectional survey. BMJ 2004;328:621–4.

10. Herwig JE, Wirtz M, Bengel J. Depression, partnership, social support, and parenting: interaction of maternal factors with behavioral problems of the child. J Affect Disord 2004;80:199–208.
11. Kim-Cohen J, Moffitt TE, Taylor A, et al. Maternal depression and children's antisocial behavior: nature and nurture effects. Arch Gen Psychiatry 2005;62:173–81.
12. Lorant V, Deliege D, Eaton W. Socioeconomic inequalities in depression: a meta-analysis. Am J Epidemiol 2003;157:98–112.
13. McFarlane J, Parker B, Morgan B. Abuse during pregnancy. A protocol for prevention and intervention. 3rd edition. New York: National March of Dimes Birth Defects Foundation; 2007.
14. Karmaliani R, Bann CM, Pirani F, et al. Diagnostic validity of two instruments for assessing anxiety and depression among pregnant women in Hyderabad, Pakistan. Health Care Women Int 2007;28:556–72.
15. Hurt H, Malmund E, Brodsky NL, et al. Exposure to violence: psychological and academic correlates in child witnesses. Arch Pediatr Adolesc Med 2001;155: 1351–6.
16. McFarlane JM, Groff JY, O'Brien JA, et al. Behaviors of children who are exposed and not exposed to intimate partner violence: an analysis of 330 black, white, and Hispanic children. Pediatrics 2003;112(3):202–7.
17. McFarlane J, Groff J, O'Brien J, et al. Behaviors of children following a randomized controlled treatment program for their abused mothers. Issues Compr Pediatr Nurs 2005;28:195–211.
18. McFarlane J, Groff J, O'Brien J, et al. Behaviors of children exposed to intimate partner violence before and one year after a treatment program for their mother. Appl Nurs Res 2005;18:7–12.
19. World Health Report. Make every child and mother count. Geneva (Switzerland): World Health Organization; 2006.
20. Ali BS, Rahber MH. The effectiveness of counseling on anxiety and depression by minimally trained counselors: a randomized controlled trial. Am J Psychother 2003;57(3):324–36.
21. Hirani S, Karmaliani R, McFarlane J, et al. Development of an economic skill building intervention to promote women's safety and child development in Karachi, Pakistan. Issues Ment Health Nurs 2010;31:82–8.
22. World Health Organization. Preventing intimate partner and sexual violence against women; taking actions and generating evidences. Geneva (Switzerland): World Health Organization; 2010.
23. Astbury J, Cabral M. Women mental health: an evidence based review. Geneva (Switzerland): World Health Organization; 2000.
24. Hussain N, Creed F, Tomenson B. Depression and social stress in Pakistan. Psychol Med 2000;30:395–402.
25. Bass J, Neugebauer R, Clougherty K, et al. Group interpersonal psychotherapy for depression in rural Uganda, 6 months outcomes. Br J Psychiatry 2006;188:567–73.
26. Davis MF. The economics of abuse: how violence perpetuates women's poverty. In: Brandwein RA, editor. Battered women, children and welfare reform: the ties that bind. Thousand Oaks (CA): Sage Publications ltd; 1999. p. 17–30.
27. Swanberg JE, Logan T, Macke C. Intimate partner violence, employment, and the workplace: consequences and future directions. Trauma Violence Abuse 2001; 6(4):286–312.
28. Tolman RM, Rosen D. Domestic violence in the lives of women receiving welfare: mental health, substance dependence and economic well being. Violence Against Women 2001;7(2):141–58.

29. Moe A, Bell MP. Abject economics: the effect of battering and violence on women's work and employability. Violence Against Women 2004;10(1):29–55.
30. World Health Organization. WHO multi-country study on women's health and domestic violence: report of initial results on prevalence, health outcomes and women's responses. Geneva (Switzerland): WHO; 2005.
31. Ford-Gilobe M, Wuest J, Varcoe C, et al. Modeling the effect of intimate partner violence and access to resources on women's health in the early years after leaving an abusive partner. Soc Sci Med 2009;68:1021–9.
32. Hirani S, Karmaliani R, McFarlane J, et al. Testing a community derived intervention to promote women's health: preliminary results of a 3-arm RCT in Karachi, Pakistan. Southern Online J Nurs Res 2010;10(3). Available at: http://snrs.org/publications/SOJNR_articles2/Vol10Num03Art06.html. Accessed August 5, 2011.
33. Garcia-Moreno C, Watts C. Violence against women: an urgent public health priority. Bull World Health Organ 2011;89(1):2.
34. Chen G, Gully SM, Eden D. General self efficacy and self esteem: toward theoretical and empirical distinction between correlated self evaluations. J Organ Behav 2004;25:375–95.
35. Scholz U, Gutierres-Dona B, Sud S, et al. Is general self efficacy a universal construct? psychometric findings from 25 countries. Eur J Psychol Assess 2002;18(3):242–51.
36. Benight CC, Harding-Taylor AS, Midboe AM, et al. Development and psychometric validation of domestic violence coping self efficacy measure (DV-CSE). J Trauma Stress 2004;17(6):505–8.
37. United Nations Population Fund and Microcredit Summit Campaign. From microfinance to macro change: integrating health education and microfinance to empower women and reduce poverty. Washington, DC: Tackett-Barbaria Design Group; 2006.
38. Dubreuil GE, Mirada CT. A model of sustainability for microcredit financial institutions. Barcelona (Spain): Departament d'Economia de l'Empresa, Universitat Autònoma de Barcelona: Emprius, 2 – 08201 Sabadell; 2005.
39. Pronyk PM, Hargeaves JR, Morduch J. Microfinance programs and better health: prospects for sub-saharan Africa. JAMA 2007;298(16):1925–7.
40. Littlefield E, Murduch J, Hashemi S. Is microfinance an effective strategy to reach the millennium development goals? Washington, DC: CGAP; 2003.
41. Setboonsarng S, Parpiev Z. Microfinance and the millennium development goals in pakistan: impact assessment using propensity score matching. Japan: Asian Development Bank Institute; 2008.
42. Lutfun N, Khan O. Impact of credit on the relative well-being of women: evidence from the Grameen Bank. IDS Bulletin 1998;29(4):31–8.
43. Schuler SR, Hashemi SM, Riley AP, et al. Credit programs, patriarchy and men's violence against women in rural Bangladesh. Soc Sci Med 1996;43(12):1729–42.

Index

Note: Page numbers of article titles are in **boldface** type.

A

Abuse, 385–493
    across the lifespan, **391–411**
        child abuse and risk factors, 398–400
        costs of, 406–408
        during pregnancy, subsequent health outcomes, 397–398
        intimate partner violence, consequences for children, 400–401
        outcomes beyond the immediate trauma, 401–406
            assessment of, 404–405
            how to stop, 405–406
            mental health consequences, 403–404
        risk factors for, 395–396
        sexual abuse, gender differences and risk factors, 396–397
        who are the victims, 392–395
    among military service members and their families, **445–455**
        family violence in military families, 448–449
        military deployment and families, 446
            research on effects o, 447–448
        sexual trauma while serving, 449–452
    bullying of adults, **423–429**
        cyberbullying, 425–426
        implications for nursing, 426–427
        in the workplace, 424–425
        interventions for, 427–428
    child, definitions, 415–417
            emotional abuse, 416
            emotional neglect, 415
            physical, 416–417
            physical neglect, 415
            sexual, 417
        education, 419–420
        epidemiology, 413–414
        factors affecting, 414–415
        implications, 420–421
        psychological issues, 418–419
        screening, 417–418
    community services for victims of, **471–476**
        children, 471–473
        elderly, 475
        intimate partners, 473–474
        prevention strategies, 475
    elder, **431–436**

Nurs Clin N Am 46 (2011) 495–502
doi:10.1016/S0029-6465(11)00081-8
0029-6465/11/$ – see front matter © 2011 Elsevier Inc. All rights reserved.

nursing.theclinics.com

Abuse (*continued*)
    aging statistics, 431–432
    community awareness, 433–434
    culture and society, 432–433
    domestic and institutional legislation, **477–484**
    health services, 433
    laws, 433
    pervasiveness, 432
    risk factors, 432
  health care, impact of interpersonal violence on, **465–470**
    child maltreatment, 466
    elder maltreatment, 468
    intimate partner violence, 467–468
    strategies to prevent interpersonal violence, 468–469
  intimate partner, relationship with depression, **437–444**
    in perpetrators of, 440–441
    intervening to reduce association between, 441–442
    link with suicide, 439
    nature of association over time, 440
    negative outcomes in women, 439
    theories regarding, 439–440
  of women in Pakistan, new interventions for, **485–495**
    challenges faced by women, 488–489
    economic skills building, 488
    group counseling, 487–488
    meeting the Millennium Development Goals for 2015 for, 486–487
    outcomes of, 489
    recommendations, 489–491
      testing microcredit, 490–491
  types of, **385–390**
    child, 385–386
    elder, 388–389
    intimate partner, 386–388
    intimate partner violence, 386–388
  workplace violence in nursing, **457–464**
    focus on verbal abuse, 457–462
Adult protective services, elder abuse legislation, **477–484**
Adults, bullying of. *See* Bullying.
Aging, statistics on, 431–432
Assessment, for abuse, considerations in, 404–405
Awareness, community, of elder abuse, 433–434

B

Bruising, in child abuse, 416
Bullying, of adults, **423–429**
    cyberbullying, 425–426
    implications for nursing, 426–427
    in the workplace, 424–425
    interventions for, 427–428
Burns, in child abuse, 416–417

C

Child abuse, 385– 386, **413–422**
   community services for victims of, 471–473
   definitions, 415–417
      emotional abuse, 416
      emotional neglect, 415
      physical, 416–417
      physical neglect, 415
      sexual, 417
   education, 419–420
   epidemiology, 413–414
   factors affecting, 414–415
   impact on health care, 466
   implications, 420–421
   psychological issues, 418–419
   risk factors for, 398– 400
   screening, 417–418
   strategies to prevent, 468–469
Children. *See also* Child abuse.
   prevalence of parental violence and consequences for, 400–401
Community awareness, of elder abuse, 433–434
Community services, for victims of interpersonal violence, **471–476**
      children, 471–473
      elderly, 475
      intimate partners, 473–474
      prevention strategies, 475
Costs, of abuse, 406–407
Counseling, group, for abused women in Pakistan, 487–488
Cultural factors, in elder abuse, 432–433
Cyberbullying, of adults, 425–426
      behaviors, 426
      consequences, 426
      reasons for, 425

D

Deployment, military, impact on families, 446–448
Depression, relationship between intimate partner abuse and, **437–444**
      in perpetrators of, 440–441
      intervening to reduce association between, 441–442
      link with suicide, 439
      nature of association over time, 440
      negative outcomes in women, 439
      theories regarding, 439–440

E

Economic skills building, as intervention for abused women in Pakistan, 488
Education, on child abuse, 419–420
Elder abuse, 388– 389, **431–436**

Elder (*continued*)
    aging statistics, 431–432
    community awareness, 433–434
    community services for victims of, 475
    culture and society, 432–433
    domestic and institutional legislation, **477–484**
        research on, 478–481
        types of, 478
        variations in, 481–483
    health services, 433
    impact on health care, 468
    laws, 433
    pervasiveness, 432
    risk factors, 432
    strategies for prevention of, 469
Electronic aggression, as means of child abuse, 386
    cyberbullying of adults, 425–426
Emotional abuse, child, definition of, 416
Emotional neglect, child, definition of, 415
Epidemiology, of child abuse, 413–414

F

Families, military, abuse in, **445–455**
    family violence, 448–449
    impact of military deployment on, 446
        research on effects of, 447–448
    sexual trauma while serving, 449–452
    violence between parents, consequences for children, 400–401

G

Gender differences, in risk factors for sexual abuse, 396–397
Group counseling, intervention for abused women in Pakistan, 487–488

H

Health care, impact of interpersonal violence on, **465–470**
    child maltreatment, 466
    elder maltreatment, 468
    intimate partner violence, 467–468
    strategies to prevent, 468–469
Health services, programs aimed at the elderly, 433

I

Interpersonal violence. *See also* Abuse.
    community services for victims of, **471–476**
        children, 471–473
        elderly, 475
        intimate partners, 473–474

prevention strategies, 475
impact on health care, **465–470**
child maltreatment, 466
elder maltreatment, 468
intimate partner violence, 467–468
strategies to prevent, 468–469
Intimate partner abuse, 386–388
between parents, consequences for children, 400–401
community services for victims of, 473–474
impact on health care, 467–468
new interventions for abused women in Pakistan, **485–495**
challenges faced by women, 488–489
economic skills building, 488
group counseling, 487–488
meeting the Millennium Development Goals for 2015 for, 486–487
outcomes of, 489
recommendations, 489–491
testing microcredit, 490–491
relationship between depression and, **437–444**
in perpetrators of, 440–441
intervening to reduce association between, 441–442
link with suicide, 439
nature of association over time, 440
negative outcomes in women, 439
theories regarding, 439–440
strategies for prevention of, 469

L

Legislation, on elder abuse, 433, **477–484**
research on, 478–481
types of, 478
variations in, 481–483

M

Men, as perpetrators of intimate partner abuse, depression in, 440–441
Mental health, consequences of abuse for, 403–404
Microcredit, as intervention to improve health of women in Pakistan, 490–491
Microfinancing. *See* Microcredit.
Military families, abuse in, **445–455**
family violence, 448–449
impact of military deployment on, 446
research on effects of, 447–448
sexual trauma while serving, 449–452
Millennium Development Goals for 2015, new interventions for abused women
in Pakistan, **485–493**
Munchausen syndrome by proxy, 415

N

National Institute for Health and Clinical Excellence (NICE), guidance on when to suspect child abuse, 419–420
Neglect, as form of child abuse, 385–386
    child, definitions of, 415
        emotional, 415
        physical, 415

O

Oppressed group behavior, due to workplace violence in nursing, 461–462
Outcomes, of abuse beyond the immediate trauma, 402–406

P

Pakistan, new interventions for abused women in, **485–495**
        challenges faced by women, 488–489
        economic skills building, 488
        group counseling, 487–488
        meeting the Millennium Development Goals for 2015 for, 486–487
        outcomes of, 489
        recommendations, 489–491
            testing microcredit, 490–491
Parents, prevalence of violence between, consequences for children, 400–401
Perpetrators, of abuse, relationship with depression in, 440–441
Physical abuse, child, definition of, 416–417
Physical neglect, child, definition of, 415
Post-traumatic stress disorder, after military deployment, 44
    after military sexual trauma, 450–452
    in children witnessing parental violence, 400–401
Pregnancy, abuse during, subsequent health outcomes, 397–398
Prevention, of interpersonal violence, 405–406
        child abuse, 468–469
        elder abuse, 469
        intimate partner violence, 469
        nurses' role in, 406
        role of community services in, 475
Psychosocial issues, in child abuse, 418–419

R

Rape, sexual trauma in the military, 448–452
Relationships, intimate partner violence, 386–388
Resources, community services for victims of interpersonal violence, **471–476**
Risk factors, for abuse, 395–400
        for child abuse, 398–399
        for elder abuse, 432
        for sexual abuse, gender differences and, 396–397

S

Screening, for child abuse, 417–418
Sexual abuse, of children, 386
    definition of, 417
  risk factors for, gender differences and, 396–397
Sexual harassment, in the military, 448–452
Sexual trauma, in the military, 448–452
Shaken baby syndrome, 386, 413–414, 417
Social networking, cyberbullying of adults, 425–426
Suicide, relationship between intimate partner abuse and, 439

T

Technology, as means of abuse, 386
Thermal injuries, in child abuse, 416–417
Trauma, sexual, in the military, 448–452

U

United Nations Development Program, meeting the Millennium Development Goals
  for 2015, **485–493**

V

Verbal abuse, in nursing workplace, 457–462
Victims, of abuse. *See also* Abuse.
  who are they, 392–395
    international prevalence studies, 392–395
Violence. *See also* Abuse.
  community services for victims of interpersonal, **471–476**
  family, in military families, 448–449
  interpersonal, community services for victims of, **471–476**
    children, 471–473
    elderly, 475
    intimate partners, 473–474
    prevention strategies, 475
  interpersonal, impact on health care, **465–470**
    child maltreatment, 466
    elder maltreatment, 468
    intimate partner violence, 467–468
    strategies to prevent, 468–469
  intimate partner, 386–388
  workplace, in nursing today, **457–464**

W

Women, abuse of. *See also* Intimate partner violence.
  during pregnancy, subsequent health outcomes of, 397–398
  in Pakistan, new interventions for, **485–495**
    challenges faced by women, 488–489

Women (*continued*)
    economic skills building, 488
    group counseling, 487–488
    meeting the Millennium Development Goals for 2015 for, 486–487
    outcomes of, 489
    recommendations, 489–491
        testing microcredit, 490–491
   intimate partner violence, 386–388
    relationship between depression and, **437–444**
Workplace violence, bullying of adults, 424–425
    behaviors, 424–425
    consequences, 425
    reasons for, 424
   in nursing, focus on verbal abuse, 457–462

United States Postal Service

Statement of Ownership, Management, and Circulation
(All Periodicals Publications Except Requestor Publications)

1. Publication Title	2. Publication Number									3. Filing Date
Nursing Clinics of North America	5	9	8	-	9	9	6	0		9/16/11

4. Issue Frequency	5. Number of Issues Published Annually	6. Annual Subscription Price
Mar, Jun, Sep, Dec	4	$135.00

7. Complete Mailing Address of Known Office of Publication (Not printer) (Street, city, county, state, and ZIP+4®)

Elsevier Inc.
360 Park Avenue South
New York, NY 10010-1710

Contact Person
Stephen Bushing
Telephone (Include area code)
215-239-3688

8. Complete Mailing Address of Headquarters or General Business Office of Publisher (Not printer)

Elsevier Inc., 360 Park Avenue South, New York, NY 10010-1710

9. Full Names and Complete Mailing Addresses of Publisher, Editor, and Managing Editor (Do not leave blank)

Publisher (Name and complete mailing address)

Kim Murphy, Elsevier, Inc., 1600 John F. Kennedy Blvd. Suite 1800, Philadelphia, PA 19103-2899

Editor (Name and complete mailing address)

Katie Hartner, Elsevier, Inc., 1600 John F. Kennedy Blvd. Suite 1800, Philadelphia, PA 19103-2899

Managing Editor (Name and complete mailing address)

Sarah Barth, Elsevier, Inc., 1600 John F. Kennedy Blvd. Suite 1800, Philadelphia, PA 19103-2899

10. Owner (Do not leave blank. If the publication is owned by a corporation, give the name and address of the corporation immediately followed by the names and addresses of all stockholders owning or holding 1 percent or more of the total amount of stock. If not owned by a corporation, give the names and addresses of the individual owners. If owned by a partnership or other unincorporated firm, give its name and address as well as those of each individual owner. If the publication is published by a nonprofit organization, give its name and address.)

Full Name	Complete Mailing Address
Wholly owned subsidiary of	4520 East-West Highway
Reed/Elsevier, US holdings	Bethesda, MD 20814

11. Known Bondholders, Mortgagees, and Other Security Holders Owning or Holding 1 Percent or More of Total Amount of Bonds, Mortgages, or Other Securities. If none, check box ☐ None

Full Name	Complete Mailing Address
N/A	

12. Tax Status (For completion by nonprofit organizations authorized to mail at nonprofit rates) (Check one)
The purpose, function, and nonprofit status of this organization and the exempt status for federal income tax purposes:
☐ Has Not Changed During Preceding 12 Months
☐ Has Changed During Preceding 12 Months (Publisher must submit explanation of change with this statement)

PS Form 3526, September 2007 (Page 1 of 3 (Instructions Page 3)) PSN 7530-01-000-9931 PRIVACY NOTICE: See our Privacy policy in www.usps.com

---

13. Publication Title			14. Issue Date for Circulation Data Below
Nursing Clinics of North America			September 2011

15. Extent and Nature of Circulation			Average No. Copies Each Issue During Preceding 12 Months	No. Copies of Single Issue Published Nearest to Filing Date
a. Total Number of Copies (Net press run)			2213	2000
b. Paid Circulation (By Mail and Outside the Mail)	(1)	Mailed Outside-County Paid Subscriptions Stated on PS Form 3541. (Include paid distribution above nominal rate, advertiser's proof copies, and exchange copies)	1260	1281
	(2)	Mailed In-County Paid Subscriptions Stated on PS Form 3541 (Include paid distribution above nominal rate, advertiser's proof copies, and exchange copies)		
	(3)	Paid Distribution Outside the Mails Including Sales Through Dealers and Carriers, Street Vendors, Counter Sales, and Other Paid Distribution Outside USPS®	293	359
	(4)	Paid Distribution by Other Classes Mailed Through the USPS (e.g. First-Class Mail®)		
c. Total Paid Distribution (Sum of 15b (1), (2), (3), and (4))		▶	1553	1640
d. Free or Nominal Rate Distribution (By Mail and Outside the Mail)	(1)	Free or Nominal Rate Outside-County Copies Included on PS Form 3541	63	50
	(2)	Free or Nominal Rate In-County Copies Included on PS Form 3541		
	(3)	Free or Nominal Rate Copies Mailed at Other Classes Through the USPS (e.g. First-Class Mail)		
	(4)	Free or Nominal Rate Distribution Outside the Mail (Carriers or other means)		
e. Total Free or Nominal Rate Distribution (Sum of 15d (1), (2), (3) and (4))		▶	63	50
f. Total Distribution (Sum of 15c and 15e)		▶	1616	1690
g. Copies not Distributed (See instructions to publishers #4 (page #3))		▶	597	310
h. Total (Sum of 15f and g)		▶	2213	2000
i. Percent Paid (15c divided by 15f times 100)			96.10%	97.04%

16. Publication of Statement of Ownership

☐ If the publication is a general publication, publication of this statement is required. Will be printed
in the December 2011 issue of this publication.   ☐ Publication not required

17. Signature and Title of Editor, Publisher, Business Manager, or Owner

Stephen R. Bushing   Date

Stephen R. Bushing —Inventory/Distribution Coordinator   September 16, 2011

I certify that all information furnished on this form is true and complete. I understand that anyone who furnishes false or misleading information on this form or who omits material or information requested on the form may be subject to criminal sanctions (including fines and imprisonment) and/or civil sanctions (including civil penalties).

PS Form 3526, September 2007 (Page 2 of 3)

Moving?

Make sure your subscription moves with you!

To notify us of your new address, find your **Clinics Account Number** (located on your mailing label above your name), and contact customer service at:

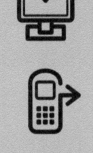

Email: journalscustomerservice-usa@elsevier.com

800-654-2452 (subscribers in the U.S. & Canada)
314-447-8871 (subscribers outside of the U.S. & Canada)

Fax number: 314-447-8029

Elsevier Health Sciences Division
Subscription Customer Service
3251 Riverport Lane
Maryland Heights, MO 63043

*To ensure uninterrupted delivery of your subscription, please notify us at least 4 weeks in advance of move.

Printed and bound by CPI Group (UK) Ltd, Croydon, CR0 4YY

03/10/2024

01040441-0011